NUTRITION DIVA'S

SECRETS FOR
A HEALTHY DIET

ALSO BY MONICA REINAGEL

The Inflammation-Free Diet Plan

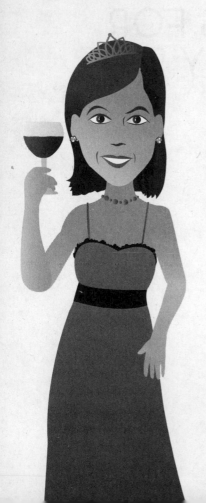

NUTRITION DIVA'S
SECRETS FOR A HEALTHY DIET

WHAT TO EAT,

WHAT TO AVOID,

AND WHAT TO STOP

WORRYING ABOUT

MONICA REINAGEL, MS, LN, CNS

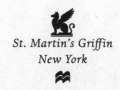

St. Martin's Griffin
New York

This book is for informational purposes only. The author has endeavored to make sure it contains reliable and accurate information. However, research on diet and nutrition is evolving and subject to interpretation, and the conclusions presented here may differ from those found in other sources. As each individual's experience may vary, readers, especially those with existing health problems, should consult their physician or health-care professional before adopting any nutritional changes based on information contained in this book. Individual readers are solely responsible for their own health-care decisions, and the author and the publisher do not accept responsibility for any adverse effects individuals may claim to experience, whether directly or indirectly, based on information contained herein.

www.stmartins.com

ISBN 978-0-312-67641-4

First Edition: March 2011

10 9 8 7 6 5 4 3 2 1

CONTENTS

PREFACE   ix

INTRODUCTION   1

PART ONE
Nutrition Diva's Guide to the Grocery Store
3

one / *Shopping the Perimeter*   5

FRESH PRODUCE   5

THE DAIRY CASE   14

EGGS   30

JUICE   32

THE MEAT DEPARTMENT   33

THE FISH COUNTER   40

two / *Stocking the Pantry*   45

GRAINS   45

PASTA   50

BREADS   54

CEREAL   56

FLOUR   58

SWEETENERS   60

SALT   68

HERBS AND SPICES   70

OILS   71

VINEGARS   77

NUTS AND SEEDS   80
DRIED FRUIT   82
DRIED BEANS   83
CANNED VEGGIES   84

three / **Packaged and Prepared Foods**   **86**

PACKAGED FOODS   87
HOW TO USE THE NUTRITION FACTS LABEL   91
MEALS TO GO   94
SWEET AND SALTY TREATS   95
BEVERAGES   98

PART TWO
The 24-Hour Diet Makeover
105

four / **Breakfast of Divas**   **107**

COFFEE, TEA, OR CAFFEINE FREE?   107
WHEN TO EAT BREAKFAST   113
WHAT TO EAT FOR BREAKFAST   115
HOW MUCH TO EAT FOR BREAKFAST   125
BREAKFAST ON THE FLY   127

five / **Power Lunch**   **129**

WHAT TO EAT FOR LUNCH   130
CARRY-OUT AND CASUAL DINING   136
HOW MUCH SHOULD YOU EAT FOR LUNCH?   141

six / **Snacking Well**   **142**

SNACKING IS OPTIONAL   142
HOW TO SNACK PROPERLY   147

seven / **Dinner Done Right**   **157**

WHAT TO EAT FOR DINNER   158
HOW TO COOK MEAT   160
HOW TO COOK VEGETABLES   1 62

GRAINS AND OTHER STARCHES   165

HOW MUCH SHOULD YOU EAT FOR DINNER?   169

EATING DINNER OUT   169

LATE-NIGHT SNACKING   172

eight / **Drinks and Desserts**   **174**

ALCOHOLIC BEVERAGES   174

SWEET STUFF   176

nine / **Curtain Calls**   **181**

NUTRITIONAL SUPPLEMENTS   181

NUTRITION AND EXERCISE   189

DIET TRENDS   191

STILL HAVE QUESTIONS?   196

NUTRITION DIVA'S RECIPES   **197**

SAMPLE MEAL PLANS   **223**

SHOPPING GUIDE   **227**

SERVING SIZE GUIDE   **232**

GUIDE TO COOKING METHODS   **233**

ACKNOWLEDGMENTS   **234**

INDEX   **235**

What Does an Opera Singer Know about Nutrition?

I WOULDN'T NORMALLY recommend taking nutrition advice from an opera singer. You should probably also be cautious about nutrition information dispensed by actresses, fashion models, health-store clerks, aerobic instructors, farmers, and TV chefs, as well. There are a lot of self-taught nutrition experts out there. I know, because I used to be one.

I originally studied music and started my career as a professional opera singer. Like most young opera singers, I supported myself with various day jobs, and one year, I got a job with a publishing company in the research department of their health division. It was a great job; I loved reading about health and nutrition and already knew a fair amount about it. Before long, I was writing short features and fillers for the publications. Within a few years, I had a pretty solid second career going as a freelance health writer. I felt like quite the expert.

That all changed, however, when I went back to school to earn a graduate degree in nutrition. I discovered that much of the information about diet and nutrition in books, magazines, newspapers, and online simply isn't true: Eating smaller meals more frequently does *not* speed your metabolism; caffeinated beverages are *not* dehydrating; swapping ground turkey for ground beef is *not* necessarily a healthier choice! There are myths, lore, and superstitions that have been repeated so many times that no one questions their basis anymore. I learned that many of the most convincing, scientific-sounding arguments about diet are based on misunderstandings or misinterpretations of the evidence. And I realized that people spend a lot of time worrying about things that simply don't matter.

When I started recording my weekly *Nutrition Diva* podcast in 2008, my plan was to offer some quick and dirty tips on eating healthy but I ended up spending a lot of time debunking myths about nutrition. In fact, it's become a bit of a mission for me. In this book, I take a closer look at a lot of popular beliefs, controversies, and urban legends, to see which ones really stand up to scientific scrutiny and which ones you can stop worrying about. I'll let you in on all the secrets about nutrition I've uncovered and demystify all of the confusing food choices you face every day—from what to put in your cart at the grocery store to what to eat for every meal and snack of the day.

The goal of the book is to help you make good choices about what you eat. But you'll quickly see that, when it comes to diet, I am neither purist nor perfectionist. The fact is, very few of us make food choices based on nutrition alone. We are also influenced by taste, cost, availability, convenience, and habit. If you're also trying to balance things like environmental impact, social and animal welfare, religious beliefs, and other factors, you'll frequently have to pick your priorities and settle for a compromise. Sometimes, you may choose to eat something not because it's good for you but because you love it. Or because someone made it for you. Or because it's the least of the available evils. I believe that any approach to diet needs to be flexible and realistic as well as science-based.

Finally, I should point out that what we know—or think we know—about nutrition is constantly evolving. Weighing how all the various aspects of diet, lifestyle, and genetics interact with, compound, or moderate one another is a complex operation. As we get more information and do more research, we sometimes have to revise our positions. That's why I don't consider this book to be the final word on diet but rather part of an ongoing conversation—one which I hope you'll be a part of.

The conversation continues through my weekly podcast and newsletter, which you'll find at www.quickanddirtytips.com. If you use Facebook or Twitter, search for *Nutrition Diva* and join me there as well!

INTRODUCTION

HEALTHFUL EATING HAS become a rather complicated business. The sheer number of decisions we have to make every day about what to eat is overwhelming. It starts the moment you wake up: Should you have coffee? Tea? Decaf? Which is the healthiest choice? It's a wonder we ever get anything else done. I'm not here to dump another book's worth of information into your overcrowded decision-making database. Rather, I'd like to help you make sense of all you've heard and read about nutrition, to sort the fact from the fiction, the good information from the bad, and the important things from the stuff that's really not worth worrying about. The idea is to make the business of eating right just a little bit simpler, a little bit saner.

At least half the battle is simply having the right stuff on hand. When healthy foods aren't readily available, most of us will take the path of least resistance, which generally leads to a fast-food restaurant, carryout place, vending machine, or the snack cupboard (you know the one I mean). So we'll begin at the grocery store, where a lot of the most important choices about food happen. We'll cover all the basic food types: fruits and vegetables; eggs, dairy, and dairy substitutes; meats and other protein sources; grains, breads, and other starches; fats and oils; and, of course, all those packaged, prepared, and frozen foods. You'll learn how (or whether) these foods fit into a healthy diet, what to look for, and what to avoid.

Choosing healthy foods is a start. But how many times have you come home from the grocery store, unloaded six bags of groceries and discovered that you don't have the ingredients for a single meal? I also have tips to ensure that you'll end up with everything you need for healthy meals throughout the week, both at home and on the road.

Once we've stocked the cupboards, the real fun begins. In the second part of the book, I'll take you through all the decisions you're likely to face in a typical day, from what to have for breakfast to whether it's ever okay to have a midnight snack. I've also included many of my favorite healthy recipes. These are the dishes that I make in my own kitchen every week—everything from on-the-go breakfasts to dinner for company. Now you'll not only know which foods are the healthiest choices at the store, you'll know what to do with them once you get them home! I've also included a few sample meal plans at the end of the book that you can use as a quick reference guide.

As the title of the book suggests, my secrets for a healthy diet can be sorted into three broad categories: what you should eat, foods to steer clear of, and things you can quit worrying about. And, really, that last category may be the most important of all. There's a lot of information out there about diet and nutrition—some of it better than others. But the more information you have, the easier it is to lose track of the things that matter most. And let's be honest: You can't pay attention to *everything*—at least, not for very long. So, in addition to helping you make the best choices at the grocery store and navigate through the many decisions you make throughout the day, my ultimate goal is to help you prioritize the things that will make the biggest difference in your health.

PART ONE
Nutrition Diva's Guide to the Grocery Store

If you want to eat better tomorrow, you need to go to the grocery store today. Unfortunately, grocery stores are not organized with your convenience, pocketbook, or health in mind. In fact, they are carefully designed to get you to spend as much as possible on foods with the greatest profit margin, which are not necessarily the foods that make you healthiest.

Another thing that makes grocery shopping daunting is the number of choices and decisions you have to make. The average grocery store has tens of thousands of options, all vying for your attention and loyalty. Even when you're hell-bent on buying healthy foods, it's easy to find yourself stymied by conflicting priorities and claims. Which is better: organic or free range? Low-fat or trans-fat free? Sugar-free or all natural? The first part of this book is for all of you stranded in aisle eight, trying to figure out whether whole grain trumps gluten-free and wondering whether resistant starches are really a good idea.

Ready to get started? Let's go shopping.

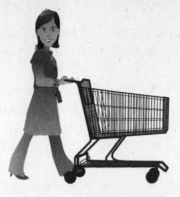

CHAPTER ONE

Shopping the Perimeter

EVERY GROCERY STORE is organized a little bit differently but you'll usually find the least-processed foods arrayed around the edges of the store and most of the processed and packaged foods in the interior aisles. "Shopping the perimeter" is a good strategy for loading up your cart with the healthiest foods. It also simplifies things a bit. After all, most of these foods have just one ingredient listed on the label or no label at all. Nonetheless, there are a still a lot of factors to weigh and a lot of decisions to make as you choose what actually goes in your cart.

FRESH PRODUCE

Most grocery stores are set up so that fresh produce is the first thing you encounter as you walk in the door. Of course, that means that your peaches and other bruiseable goods inevitably end up on the bottom of the cart, crushed underneath a forty-pound bag of dog food. On the other hand, starting with the fresh fruits and vegetables presents an opportunity: The more you pile into your cart here, the less room there will be for all of those treacherous items over in the snack food aisle. Unfortunately, most people tend to under-shop in the produce department. They toss a head of lettuce, a stalk of broccoli, and a bag of carrots into the cart and move on. But hang on a minute: We're supposed to be eating five servings of veggies a day. If you're shopping for two people and you go to the store twice a week, then you should have something like thirty-five servings of veggies in your cart! Of course, you probably eat some percentage of your meals on the road. But you get my point.

As a general rule, vegetables should take up at least a third (or even half) of the real estate on your plate. Logically, this means that veggies should take up at least a third of your grocery cart.

Why Is Produce So Expensive?

Although fresh fruits and vegetables are the most nutritious items you'll find in the grocery store, they are also some of the most expensive. Or at least they *seem* expensive. But are they really as costly as we think? I've noticed that many people (myself included) seem to have a double standard when it comes to these things. Those gorgeous red bell peppers, for example, seem kind of expensive at $1.50 each. And yet we think nothing of tossing a three-dollar bag of potato chips into the cart. The cost per serving works out to be about the same. But the chips contribute virtually nothing to your diet except unhealthy fats, sodium, and empty calories. A single red pepper, on the other hand, provides a more than day's worth of vitamins A and C, and a decent amount of fiber, folate, and vitamin E. Talk about a good return on your investment!

If produce still seems expensive, just remember that eating more vegetables lowers your risk of disease and can reduce your health-care expenses in the future. Finally, remember that veggies should take up about a third of your grocery cart—so it's okay if they take up a third of your grocery bill as well.

The Best Choices in Produce

Certain fruits and vegetables have a reputation for being extra nutritious. They're either particularly good sources of certain nutrients, or they've been found to contain uniquely beneficial compounds. Kale is an excellent source of calcium, for example, and grapes are rich in resveratrol, an antioxidant that is thought to protect your heart. The pigments that make plants green, orange, or purple seem to be particularly beneficial to humans, which is why there is often a lot of emphasis on colorful fruits and vegetables like carrots, sweet potatoes, leafy greens, and berries. But there's also plenty of nutrition in foods like white mushrooms, cauliflower, garlic, and onions.

There are a few nutritional slackers in the produce section as well. Just-picked corn on the cob or freshly dug new potatoes are among the short-lived joys of summer. But on the whole, starchy vegetables like corn and potatoes are on the low end of the nutritional spectrum. In the table on page 8, you'll find some of the most nutritious fruits and vegetable choices. But don't hesitate to play the field. Because the various families of plants have such different nutrient profiles, I think you get more benefit from eating a wide variety of fruits and vegetables than you do from eating the same one or two "superfoods" day after day. When shopping for vegetables, try to include at least one thing from each of the following groups:

GREEN—(lettuce, spinach, kale, Swiss chard,
   beet and mustard greens, etc.)

RED/ORANGE—(tomatoes, carrots, sweet potatoes,
   winter squash, red peppers)

CRUCIFEROUS—(cabbage, broccoli, cauliflower, brussels sprouts)

PODS—(peas, green beans, snowpeas, etc.)

STINKERS—(onions, scallions, shallots, garlic)

Produce Power Picks

VEGETABLES	FRUITS
bell peppers (especially red, yellow, orange)	apricots (fresh)
cabbage family (broccoli, brussels sprouts, cabbage, cauliflower)	berries (all kinds)
	cantaloupe
carrots	cherries
fresh herbs	citrus
garlic, onions	grapes (especially red or purple)
leafy greens (arugula, collards, kale, Swiss chard)	kiwi
mushrooms	pomegranate
sweet potatoes	
tomatoes	
winter squash	

Getting the Most for Your Money

Another way to get the most nutrition for your money is to look for produce that's in season and grown close to where you live. Local, seasonal produce generally spends less time in transit and storage, where nutrients can fade. Keeping it local also keeps costs down, because you're paying for less fuel. If you garden or go to farmer's markets, you've probably got a good idea what grows at various times of the year in your area. If you don't, you may have no idea whether asparagus is a spring or fall vegetable. See "What's in Season?" on the next page for a quick guide to what's in season when.

THE QUICK AND DIRTY SECRET

Produce that's local and in season offers the best value, nutritionally and otherwise.

What's in Season?

	SPRING	SUMMER	LATER SUMMER/ EARLY FALL	LATE FALL/ WINTER
fruits	rhubarb	apricots berries cantaloupe nectarines peaches watermelon	apples pears	clementines grapefruit lemon lime orange pomegranate tangerine
vegetables	asparagus beets carrots mesclun mix and other baby greens onions peas radishes scallions	beans chard corn cucumbers eggplant garlic lettuce potatoes squash tomatoes zucchini	artichokes beans beets broccoli cabbage carrots cauliflower chard garlic kale leeks lettuce onions pumpkins turnips winter squash	beets broccoli Brussels sprouts cabbage carrots endive kale and other hardy greens parsnips radicchio turnips rutabaga winter squash

Note: Growing seasons and harvest dates vary greatly according to the local climate. For specifics according to location, check out the online guide at sustainabletable.org: http://www.sustainabletable.org/shop/eatseasonal/

Are Organic Vegetables Worth the Money?

If you're on a budget, you may be wondering whether it's worth paying a premium for organic produce, which is grown without synthetic fertilizers, pesticides, or herbicides. To be honest, if it were only about nutrient content, I think I'd have a hard time making the case that organics are worth the extra money. By and large, you get just as many vitamins and minerals from conventional produce as you do from organics. (See "Is Organic Produce More Nutritious?" on page 11.)

The case for organics has more to do with what's not in them.

Conventionally grown products can contain pesticide and herbicide residues—toxic chemicals that accumulate in the body over time. Agricultural chemicals also end up in the water supply, where you may be exposed to them even if you don't eat conventional produce. Exposure to these chemicals may contribute to cancer risk (especially in children) and reproductive problems, such as infertility and miscarriages.

Because organic fruits and vegetables are grown without synthetic fertilizers and pesticides, they reduce the chemical burden on the environment, wildlife, and consumers like you. Whenever the organic option is even close to the same cost as conventional, choose organic! Not only does it keep harmful chemicals out of your body but it helps keep them out of the environment—which helps everyone.

When organic options are either not available or are too expensive, you can still minimize your exposure to pesticides by knowing which fruits and vegetables have the highest pesticide residues. Of commonly eaten fruits and vegetables, these twelve foods have the highest pesticide residues: peaches, bell peppers, nectarines, cherries, grapes (imported), lettuce, apples, celery, strawberries, pears, spinach, and potatoes.

According to analysis done by the Environmental Working Group, avoiding the so-called dirty dozen can reduce your pesticide exposure by 90 percent. This list can help you decide when it might be worth it to either pay the organic premium or choose something else instead. If you or your kids eat an apple every day, for example, you might want to consider buying organic apples or substituting a conventionally grown fruit with lower chemical residues, such as oranges. The EWG has a nifty wallet guide that you can print out and take with you to remind you which foods are on the Dirty Dozen list. You'll find it on their Web site at http://foodnews.org.

I think it's worth doing what you can to reduce exposure to pesticides—especially in young kids. (Experts estimate that 50 percent of our lifetime exposure to pesticides occurs before we are five years old!) Ultimately, however, you need to keep the relative risks in per-

spective. Epidemiologists believe that healthier diet and lifestyle habits—such as eating more fresh fruits and vegetables—could prevent
one-third to one-half of all cancer cases, despite the fact that this
might increase exposure to pesticide residues.

Peeling foods like apples, peaches, and potatoes will also remove
some of the pesticide residue, but at the cost of some nutrients. Washing produce thoroughly in a solution of equal parts white vinegar and
water can also help reduce pesticide residues. It also removes dirt
and bacteria—which is why organic produce should be washed the
same way.

THE QUICK AND DIRTY SECRET

Don't let fears about pesticides keep you from eating fruits and
vegetables. If organic produce isn't available or affordable, the
benefits of eating fruits and vegetables still far outweigh the risks
of pesticide exposure.

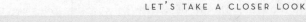

LET'S TAKE A CLOSER LOOK

Is Organic Produce More Nutritious?

Because we place such a high value these days on doing things naturally, we expect that organic vegetables should be more nutritious
than nonorganic ones. In fact, the research has shown mixed results.
Some studies have found higher levels of nutrients in organic vegetables; others have found that organic produce was no more nutritious than regular vegetables. A few even found that conventional
produce had more nutrients. In a review of 162 different studies on
the nutritional content of organic versus conventional produce, Brit-
ish researchers recently concluded that that organics are, on average, no more nutritious than regular vegetables.

Because nutrients begin to fade as soon as produce is picked,
how fresh the produce is has a much bigger impact on the nutritional

content than whether it was conventionally or organically grown. A conventionally raised tomato that you buy at a roadside stand the day after it is picked is almost certain to contain more nutrients than an organically raised tomato that was picked two weeks ago and shipped to your grocery store from another continent.

THE QUICK AND DIRTY SECRET

Buying organic reduces your exposure to pesticides but doesn't have a big effect on the nutritional quality.

Don't Forget the Fresh Herbs

Like virtually all leafy green plants, herbs are quite nutritious. But ounce for ounce, fresh herbs like oregano, rosemary, parsley, and basil are among the most nutritious greens you can find. Compared with the same amount of lettuce, raw parsley gives you three times as much vitamin A, four times as much calcium, five times as much iron, seventeen times as much vitamin K, and forty-four times as much vitamin C. Similarly, the total antioxidant capacity of fresh oregano is eight times higher than spinach. Herbs are also very rich in a wide range of disease-fighting phytochemicals. Of course, we tend to eat lettuce and spinach by the handful and parsley and oregano by the pinch, so it's not exactly a fair comparison. But you get the idea. Herbs are a very concentrated source of both flavor *and* nutrition. In both respects, a little goes a long way so don't leave the produce aisle before putting some fresh herbs in your cart.

Frozen Fruits and Vegetables

When fresh, local produce is limited or pricey, frozen fruits and vegetables can be nutritious and budget-friendly alternatives. Some nutrients are lost in processing, of course. But because they are harvested at their nutritional peak and processed immediately—often right next to the fields, frozen vegetables can actually be more nutritious than fresh produce that travels halfway around the world to your local grocery store. Frozen berries, broccoli, green beans, and winter squash are all nutritious choices that freeze well.

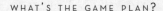

Your Shopping Game Plan for Produce

Buy enough. The goal is to eat about two-and-a-half cups of vegetables and two cups of fruit every day. To be sure you're sufficiently stocked, do a quick calculation of the number of people you're shopping for, the number of days until your next shopping trip, and the number of meals you'll be preparing at home (don't forget about lunches and snacks you'll be taking to school and work).

Choose some that you can eat raw. Some nutrients, such as vitamin C, are lost when you cook vegetables. Others, such as lycopene, are made more available. To get the best of both, buy some vegetables to cook (beans, broccoli, squash, and greens) and some to eat raw (salad greens, crudites). I'll have tips in chapter 7 for minimizing nutrient losses when cooking vegetables.

Include some things that carry well. Having portable options like apples, oranges, bananas, baby carrots, snow peas, and radishes makes it easier to grab fruits and vegetables for healthier snacks and to toss them into lunches.

Think shelf-life. Some produce keeps better than others. Berries, ripe melons or peaches, fresh herbs, and delicate lettuces may keep only a day or two. Apples, citrus fruit, kale, winter squash, and green beans will keep much longer. If it will be several days before you will be shopping again, make sure at least some of the produce you buy is more durable—and plan to consume the short-lived stuff first.

Plan meals on the fly. Choose your produce based on whatever's freshest, most inviting, and a good value. But as you make your selections, consider what you might serve with each item and whether you need to add any additional items for those meals or recipes. For example, is fennel on sale this week? Braised Fennel (recipe on page 212) makes the perfect accompaniment for grilled or baked fish. So, grab some fresh lemons before you leave the produce section and make a mental note to stop by the fish counter. (Or, if you're as easily distracted as I am at the grocery store, make an actual note on your shopping list!)

THE DAIRY CASE

When you get to the dairy section, the first decision you need to make is whether to eat dairy at all. Dairy products are a major source of vitamin D in the American diet—which is ironic, because dairy products contain very little vitamin D naturally. Milk and other dairy products are fortified with vitamin D in order to help prevent deficiency. They are also good sources of absorbable calcium and high-quality protein.

If you are allergic to dairy, are lactose intolerant, don't care for it, or don't consume animal products, you can get vitamin D, calcium, and protein from other sources. Nondairy alternatives, such as soy and rice milk, are often fortified with calcium and vitamin D. Canned fish, such as sardines and salmon, are naturally rich in protein, calcium, and vitamin D. Vegetables like broccoli and dark leafy greens are also good sources of calcium, and your body makes vitamin D when your skin is exposed to natural sunlight.

THE QUICK AND DIRTY SECRET

Dairy foods can be a good source of protein, calcium, and vitamin D but they are not essential to a healthy diet.

Are Dairy Products Bad for You?

Clearly, dairy is not essential to a healthy diet. But there are many who claim that dairy products are actually bad for you. I think most of these charges are exaggerated. If you don't like dairy or don't want to eat it, that's fine. If, on the other hand, you enjoy dairy but are nervous about things you've heard, perhaps I can set your mind at ease.

DOES DAIRY CAUSE CANCER?—*The China Study* by Colin Campbell has convinced many people that dairy products cause cancer, particularly breast cancer. Although the book is very compelling, the actual evidence is a little skimpy. Campbell bases his case on a single study that found low rates of breast cancer in a rural Chinese population that ate very little dairy, plus laboratory studies on rats and cells in petri dishes. However, dozens of more recent human studies in the United States and Europe have found absolutely no link between dairy consumption and breast cancer (or other cancers). In fact, several studies found that women who consumed more dairy had a slightly *lower* incidence of breast cancer.

DOES DAIRY CAUSE OSTEOPOROSIS?—Similarly, many folks like to point out that nations with the highest dairy consumptions have the highest rates of osteoporosis. This, however, does not remotely prove that eating dairy products causes osteoporosis. As statistics students repeatedly have drummed into their heads: correlation is not causation! My dog always seems to be standing right next to me whenever I drop cheese on the floor. However, the dog's presence does not *cause* me to drop cheese (unless I'm just being a softie). Many factors contribute to osteoporosis: inadequate intake of protein, vitamin D, calcium, magnesium, and other minerals; excessive intake of protein, sodium, or phosphates; as well as nondietary factors like exercise, genetics, age, and smoking. Dairy products provide vitamin D, calcium, and magnesium, are low in sodium and phosphates, and are neutral in terms of the rest. In other words, high dairy intake is the least likely explanation for high osteoporosis rates.

IS IT UNNATURAL TO CONSUME DAIRY PRODUCTS?—Another argument against eating dairy products is that humans are, by and large, the only animals to drink the milk of other species and to drink milk at all past infancy. To some, this is proof that consuming dairy is a bad idea. I've never found this argument particularly convincing. Humans are also the only animals to cover their bodies with clothing or to cook and preserve their foods—both of which enabled our species to survive and thrive. More to the point, humans are the only animals that have learned to keep livestock animals for milk. By grazing animals on land that is untillable, farmers can convert grass to high-quality protein and absorbable calcium—a pretty useful trick. Perhaps that's why some branches of the human family tree evolved to continue to produce lactase (the milk-digesting enzyme) into adulthood.

Should You Buy Organic Dairy?

Organic milk will cost you a dollar or so more per half gallon than conventional milk. What are you getting for the extra moola? First, you are getting milk from cows that were fed organic feed and/or grazed on fields that were not treated with synthetic chemicals. Organic dairy products are free of these chemicals. However, you should know that pesticide residues are generally not found in milk from conventionally raised cows, either.

Secondly, dairy cows that are not organically raised are often treated with a hormone (rBST) to increase milk production. Some worry that these hormones may have harmful effects on humans who consume the milk. So far, however, investigations have failed to turn up any evidence to support these fears. A stronger argument can be made that the use of the hormones causes undue stress and suffering for the cows. Hormones are not used to stimulate milk production in organic dairy cows—which may improve the cow's quality of life. However, it does not mean that organic milk is hormone-free. Although organic cows aren't given hormones, they still produce their own. If you're concerned about consuming bovine hormones, you're better off with a dairy alternative.

The last difference between organic and conventional milk is that organic cows are not given antibiotics. It's important to understand that the antibiotics given to conventional dairy cows do not end up in their milk. However, the routine use of antibiotics in livestock promotes antibiotic resistance, which is a serious problem for everyone, whether or not they drink milk. Buying organic helps to cut down on the use of antibiotics.

How do organic and conventional milk compare nutritionally? Both contain the same amount of protein, fat, calories, and calcium. If the organic cows are primarily pasture raised (which is not guaranteed), their milk will likely have more vitamins E, A, and other nutrients, especially in the summertime when the pastures are verdant.

Many consumers are convinced that organic milk simply tastes better. Or at least it used to. Unfortunately, most of the biggest organic milk producers now use ultrapasteurization to extend the shelf-life of their products. By heating the milk to about 260 degrees Fahrenheit (regular pasteurization is at 160 degrees F), they can triple the shelf-life of the milk, but at the expense of the flavor. To me, ultrapasteurized milk has a slightly flat, stale taste. Your best bet for organic milk that has not been ultrapasteurized is to find a small, local dairy. You can search for local vendors at LocalHarvest.org.

THE QUICK AND DIRTY SECRET

Nutritionally speaking, organic milk is comparable to conventional milk. But buying organic reduces the use of antibiotics in livestock, which is definitely better for you and the environment.

Should You Buy Reduced-fat Dairy Products?

The big government and public health agencies strongly recommend that you choose low-fat dairy products for two reasons. First, they are lower in saturated fat. Up until recently, saturated fat consumption was thought to contribute to heart disease. Lately, however, the connection between saturated fat and heart disease has become a matter of some debate. In 2010, an analysis of several large, long-term research studies found that people who ate the *least* saturated fat had the same risk of heart disease and stroke as the people who ate the *most* saturated fat. That's certainly food for thought—but the question is far from settled.

Saturated fat aside, low-fat dairy products are also lower in calories. As two out of three Americans—and a growing percentage of those in other countries as well—are now overweight, cutting a few calories here and there doesn't seem like such a bad idea and lower-fat dairy products is one easy way to do it. Switching from whole-fat to low-fat dairy products saves you about 40 calories per serving. If you have three servings per day, that single change could add up to twelve pounds a year. Lower-fat dairy products also give you a bit more protein and calcium per serving.

How Many Calories Are You Saving?

Whole (3.25% fat) = 146 calories per cup
Reduced-fat (2% fat) = 122 calories per cup
Low-fat (1% fat) = 102 calories per cup
Skim (0% fat) = 83 calories per cup

Each step down the fat ladder saves you about 20 calories per serving.

If you're used to drinking whole milk, skim milk might taste thin and watery to you—and that's no fun. But most people find that they can get used to and even come to prefer lower-fat products. The trick is to reduce the amount of fat gradually. Replace your whole milk with 2 percent milk or, if that's too drastic, you can even mix whole milk and 2 percent together at first, gradually reducing the proportion of whole milk. You can use the same trick to transition from 2 percent to 1 percent milk.

How low should you go? If you enjoy skim milk, that's fine. You'll also find brands of skim (fat-free) milk that have been enhanced to make them creamier. It's done by adding dried milk powder to skim milk, a trick that gives the milk more body but doesn't add any fat. It also increases the protein and calcium—as well as the calories—by about 30 percent. You'll also pay about 50 percent more for enhanced milk.

Personally, I prefer reduced- and low-fat to completely fat-free dairy products because I think a wee bit of fat makes them better-tasting and more satisfying.

THE QUICK AND DIRTY SECRET

Choosing low-fat dairy products is an easy way to cut calories (and get a bit more protein and calcium per serving) but you don't necessarily need to go completely fat-free.

Is Lactose-free Milk Better for You?

Lactose-free milk is treated with an enzyme that breaks down the natural sugars (lactose) found in milk. About 10 percent of the population does not produce this enzyme on their own and therefore has difficulty digesting milk. (You are much more likely to be lactose intolerant if you are of African, Asian, or Native American heritage.) If you are lactose intolerant, lactose-free dairy products may allow you to eat dairy products without unpleasant digestive symptoms. If you're not, there is no nutritional advantage to buying lactose-free products.

How Do You Make Fat-free Cream?

Reduced-fat milk or yogurt is one thing but when I see fat-free dairy products like sour cream, half-and-half, or cream cheese, I get suspicious. These foods are, by definition, high in fat. How can fat-free sour cream be "rich and creamy"? There's no such thing as a free lunch…and it turns out there's no such thing as fat-free cream, either. Check the ingredient label on these products and you're likely to find a long list of gelatins, gums, starches, syrups, oils, and other additives used to create a creamy consistency in fat-free products. Some of these are fairly harmless. Agar, for example, is a commonly used thickener derived from seaweed. Guar gum comes from a type of bean. But I'd rather you ate your beans and/or seaweed in a salad than in your coffee. In general, I suggest you stick to products without such elaborate ingredient lists—even if it means a gram or two of fat in your sour cream or cream cheese.

THE QUICK AND DIRTY SECRET

Choose low-fat dairy products with a gram or two of fat over fat-free products with elaborate ingredient lists.

Nondairy Milks

If you don't want to consume dairy products, there are all kinds of alternative "milks" made from soy, rice, and various nuts and grains. All are vegan and lactose-free. But do alternative milks offer any nutritional advantages over cow's milk? There are pros and cons for each type of milk, so it really depends on what your nutritional priorities are.

SOYMILK—If you're looking for protein, soymilk is your best bet. It's the only one that's comparable to cow's milk, providing between 8 and 11 grams of protein per cup. Soy protein also has beneficial effects on cholesterol levels and helps keep your bones strong. On the other hand, soy is a very common allergen. Even if you're not allergic to it, there are a few reasons that you don't want to overdo it with soy. (I'll get to that in a minute). I suggest that you keep it to no more than three servings of soy per day. If you eat a lot of other soy-based foods, you might want to choose a different type of milk.

HEMP—A relative new-comer on the alternative milk scene, hemp milk's big claim to fame is that it is an excellent source of omega-3 fats—a nutrient that most of us could use more of in our diets. Hemp milk is relatively low in protein, however, so if you're looking for a good source of protein you'll want to choose another kind.

ALMOND—If you're counting calories, almond milk tends to be lower in calories and sugar than most of the other nondairy milks. However, it is also fairly low in protein.

OAT—Oat milk offers fiber as well as a moderate amount of protein—about half as much per serving as cow's or soy milk. However, it is on the higher end in terms of sugar and calories.

RICE—Rice milk is one you're least likely to be allergic to but it's probably the least nutritious milk alternative. It's the lowest in protein and tends to be higher in sugar and calories.

See the following box for tips on which nondairy "milk" might be the best choice for you. If you've got room in the fridge, there's no reason you can't mix and match milks—and benefits.

Best Choices in Nondairy Milk

Higher in protein: soy milk
Lower in sugar/calories: almond milk
Higher in fiber: soy milk, oat milk
Higher in omega-3: hemp

Nondairy milks are not naturally high in calcium or vitamin D, but some brands are fortified to make them comparable to cow's milk as a source of these nutrients. Check the label to see exactly what you're getting—especially if you're counting on these foods to help you meet your requirements. But nutrients aren't the only things that get added to nondairy milks. Most also contain added sugar, salt, and other things to improve the flavor. Sometimes, they improve the flavor so much that they actually turn it into a dessert.

Even the plain unflavored versions can contain as much as 20 grams of added sugars per serving. That's five teaspoons of sugar in every cup. Sodium may range from 25 to 180 milligrams per serving. Check the nutrition facts labels and look for brands that keep the sugar to 12 grams or less and the sodium to no more than 100 miligrams per serving, which is similar to the amount of natural sugar and sodium present in cow's milk.

THE QUICK AND DIRTY SECRET

Dairy-free milk should contain no more than 12 grams of sugar and 100 milligrams of sodium per serving.

LET'S TAKE A CLOSER LOOK

Is Soy Dangerous?

Soy is a fairly common allergen and should obviously be avoided by anyone with a soy allergy. But there are claims that soy is dangerous for everyone else, as well. Here is a closer look at some of these charges:

Could soy cause breast cancer? Soy contains compounds called isoflavones, which are very similar to the hormone estrogen. In fact, isoflavones are also called *phytoestrogens*, which means "plant estrogens." It's thought that phytoestrogens may help *prevent* tumor formation in healthy breast tissue, and might also help protect against bone loss and alleviate hot flashes. However, in women *with* breast cancer, there is concern that phytoestrogens might promote the growth of estrogen-sensitive tumors. Just in case, those with breast cancer should avoid soy. However, there's no evidence that soy causes cancer.

Should men avoid soy? It's been suggested that excessive soy consumption might affect fertility or sexual function in men. However, studies have shown that moderate consumption of soy milk or other forms of soy protein (two to five servings per day) does not affect testosterone levels in men. In fact, soy appears to reduce the level of certain types of estrogen in men, which may have protective effects against prostate cancer. Moderate soy intake has also been shown to reduce risk factors for heart disease. Finally, keep in mind that men have been eating soy and plenty of it for generations in Asia and have not experienced population-wide fertility issues. In fact, the population of Asia enjoys lower rates of heart disease and prostate cancer.

Is soy formula bad for babies? There are similar concerns that giving soy formula to babies might affect their development. The idea is that babies, both in the womb and after birth, are extremely sensitive to hormones and that phytoestrogens might affect their development. I think we can all agree that human breast milk is by far the optimal food for babies. Sometimes, however, breast-feeding is not an option and soy formula can be a lifesaver for babies who have an allergy to cow's milk. Though there is no hard and fast evidence that soy formula causes problems, many pediatricians agree that it's best not to give soy formula to babies unless you absolutely have to—just in case.

Does soy disrupt thyroid function? Another widely repeated charge against soy is that it disrupts thyroid function. In fact, studies overwhelmingly show that it has minimal, if any, effect on thyroid function in human beings, except if they are deficient in iodine. Iodine deficiency is rare, thanks to our iodized salt supply.

Does soy contain antinutrients? Soybeans contain phytates, which can impair your ability to absorb certain nutrients. That is not unique to soy, however. Spinach contains compounds called oxalates, which do the same thing. In the context of a nutritious diet, a moderate amount of soy is unlikely to cause nutritional deficiencies. Fermenting soy removes or deactivates many of the so-called antinutrients. Fermented soy foods include miso, tempeh, natto, and soy sauce.

THE QUICK AND DIRTY SECRET

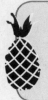

Moderate intake of soy protein may offer some health benefits, but more is not necessarily better. Two or three servings of soy foods a day is enough to provide benefit but unlikely to cause problems in healthy adults. And, as with most foods, the less processed, the better.

Yogurt and Other Friends with Benefits

Yogurt, buttermilk, and kefir are a special category of dairy. Like milk, they are all good sources of protein and calcium, but these cultured products offer an added bonus. The friendly bacteria found in these foods set up housekeeping in your gut, where they do all kinds of good things for you: They help digest your food and produce certain vitamins. They keep the lining of your intestines slick and shiny. Most of all, they make it harder for unfriendly bacteria to take hold and make you sick.

Our digestive systems work best when they have a healthy population of beneficial bacteria on board. Eating yogurt or kefir on a regular basis is a good way to help your personal population thrive. Here are some things to look for when selecting cultured foods:

LIVE CULTURES—Look for the brands that specify that they contain "live and active cultures." But don't bother paying extra for fancy brands that are supposed to be specially formulated to promote digestive health. You get the same benefits from regular yogurt.

Freezing does not kill beneficial bacteria. In fact, it preserves them in a state of suspended animation until you eat them, at which point they warm up and resume their regular helpful activities, like fending off harmful bacteria, aiding with digestion, and producing certain vitamins. So you still get all the benefits of yogurt in a frozen-fruit smoothie. But most of the frozen yogurt you buy at the grocery store or ice cream store is heat-processed before it is frozen, which destroys the beneficial bacteria. If you can find a brand that specifies that it contains "live and active cultures," you've hit the jackpot. Just keep in mind that frozen yogurt usually has a significant amount of sugar.

PLAIN, UNSWEETENED—Sweetened yogurts that you buy in the store contain so much sugar that I'm not sure you can still consider them healthy choices. Ironically, the ones with the fruit in them, which you would think might be healthier, have the most sugar. Artificially sweetened yogurts may seem at first like a healthier choice, but take a look at the ingredient list: artificial sweeteners, gelatin, colors, and assorted chemicals. Plain, unsweetened yogurt is your best choice. You can sweeten it with pureed fruit or a small amount of honey or maple syrup. As a compromise, if you really prefer sweetened yogurt, lemon- , vanilla- , and coffee-flavored yogurts are usually lower in sugar than other fruit flavors.

LOW-FAT—Low-fat yogurt has 30 percent fewer calories and 20 percent more protein than regular yogurt. Fat-free doesn't offer much additional advantage. Plus, the less fat yogurt contains, the more tart it tends to taste. So, you may find that you need a lot less sweetener if you get low-fat yogurt instead of fat-free yogurt.

THE QUICK AND DIRTY SECRET

Lemon, vanilla, and coffee-flavored yogurts have about 25 percent less sugar than most fruit-flavored yogurts.

Is Greek-style Yogurt Better for You?

Greek-style yogurt is thicker and many people also find it milder-tasting than regular yogurt. It's made by straining some of the whey out of the yogurt. A quart of milk produces four cups of regular yogurt, but only two-and-a-half to three cups of Greek-style yogurt. (That's one reason it's so much more expensive.) Because it's more concentrated, low-fat and fat-free Greek yogurt provides up to twice as much protein as the same amount of regular low-fat or fat-free yogurt, along with a few extra calories. Watch out for "classic" or full-fat Greek yogurt, though. It contains as much fat as premium ice cream—and almost twice as many calories as regular full-fat yogurt. And if you're looking for a good source of calcium, stick with regular yogurt, which is quite a bit higher in calcium than Greek-style. (Apparently, some of the calcium is strained off with the whey.)

THE QUICK AND DIRTY SECRET

Low-fat or fat-free Greek-style yogurt is higher in protein but lower in calcium than regular yogurt.

Cheese

Cheese is basically milk in miniature. The nutritional profile of each cheese will depend in part on what kind of milk or cream it was made with. For example, heavy cream can be transformed into super-rich triple-cream brie that contains 200 calories per bite. Low-fat milk can be made into part-skim ricotta that's 200 calories per cup.

The calorie density also depends on how much liquid is removed. A cup of liquid milk—and all the calories it contains—can be reduced to a half-cup of soft cheese or pressed into two cubic inches of hard cheese. As a general rule, the harder and drier the cheese, the more calories per ounce it will contain. Many people are surprised to learn than an ounce of aged cheddar has more calories than an ounce of ripe Camembert.

On average, a serving of cheese will provide 100 calories, 10 percent of your protein needs, and between 10 and 20 percent of your daily calcium requirements.

For a few picks that beat the averages, see the box below. But for the cheeses that you're likely to find at the grocery store, the differences are minor enough that you can afford to enjoy some variety.

Best Picks in the Cheese Department

Higher in protein and calcium: Gruyere, Parmesan, Gouda, cottage cheese

Lower in fat and calories: part-skim ricotta, mozzarella, feta, goat, cottage cheese

Lower in sodium: Camembert, Swiss

Note: *If you're watching sodium, avoid cottage cheese, blue cheese, Gouda, feta, and Parmesan.*

WHAT'S THE GAME PLAN?

Your Shopping Game Plan for Dairy

If you include dairy in your diet, two or three servings per person per day is a good rule of thumb for shopping. A serving is one cup (8 ounces) of milk or yogurt, a half-cup (4 ounces) of ricotta or cottage cheese, and one ounce of hard cheese. Here are some other considerations that can make meal-planning easier:

Pourable Milk and nondairy milks all have a relatively long shelf life, so buy enough to cover your household's cooking and drinking needs until your next shopping trip. But check expiration dates to avoid buying milk that's nearing the end of its shelf life.

Portable Yogurt, cottage cheese, string cheese, and individual serving cheeses (such as Babybel) are convenient for snacks and lunches at work or school. You can save some money and reduce waste by buying large containers of yogurt and cottage cheese and spooning it into smaller, reusable containers to take with you.

Practical Keeping a couple of versatile cheeses on hand also makes it easier to whip up last-minute meals. Particularly handy options include feta cheese to crumble on salads, mozzarella to sprinkle on a homemade pizza or bowl of minestrone, a brick of cheddar or Monterey for quick quesadillas or to top a frittata. (See, for example, my recipe for Leftover Vegetable Frittata on page 200.)

Butter and Margarine

Most people like to keep a little butter or margarine on hand. Which is the better choice? The main case against butter is that it's high in saturated fat—but as I mentioned earlier, saturated fat may not be the artery-clogger we once thought it was. On the plus side, butter has its incomparable flavor going for it. It's also a very simple, natural product, made from cream and (sometimes) salt. Margarine is made from vegetable oils and usually has a considerably longer ingredient list. Flavorings, colorings, stabilizers, and texturizers are added to make it look and taste more like butter. (Some people find this disguise more convincing than others.)

If you choose margarine, read the label carefully and avoid any product that contains partially hydrogenated oils, esters, or esterified oils in its ingredient list. These ingredients signal the presence of trans fats or their equally dangerous (but lesser-known) cousins, interesterified fats. You don't want either one in your body.

These days, margarines are also likely to contain ingredients that promise various health benefits. If you like the idea of food that works a little harder, you can find butterlike spreads tricked out with phytosterols and omega-3 fatty acids—nutrients that can help lower cholesterol and promote heart health. Be prepared to pay a premium. For me, it's no contest: I'd rather stick with butter and get my phytosterols and omega-3 fatty acids from foods that contain them naturally, such as nuts and fish.

Spreads with added omega-3 fats or plant esters may offer additional benefits; but avoid spreads made with hydrogenated and/or esterified oils.

Reduced-fat Spreads

Butter and margarine are both nearly pure fat, which means they are relatively high in calories—about 100 calories per tablespoon. You'll also find "light" and "reduced-fat" spreads in the dairy case. These are made by whipping water, air, milk solids, and any number of other dairy and nondairy ingredients into butter or margarine. These products can help save you a few calories. So can simply using less regular butter or margarine. If you do opt for a reduced-fat spread, read the label carefully to avoid trans and interesterified fats. Also, be aware that replacing butter with a reduced-fat butter replacement in a recipe may lead to disappointing results, especially when baking.

KITCHEN TIP

Make Your Own Healthy Butter Spread

Butter stays fresher when kept in the refrigerator, but cold butter can really tear up a piece of toast. Make your own spreadable butter by blending two sticks of softened butter with ½ cup of canola or extra-light olive oil in your blender until it's smooth. (Add a pinch of salt if the butter is unsalted.) This all-natural butter blend tastes like butter but is lower in saturated fats, higher in heart-healthy monounsaturated fats, and—best of all—is spreadable straight out of the fridge. (Note that it's not lower in fat or calories than regular butter.)

What about Spray Butter?

Imitation butter sprays are applied with an atomizer, which makes it possible to add very small amounts of these products to your food. Although the "Nutrition Facts" label may say that a butter-flavored spray contains zero fat and calories, this is simply a sleight of hand due to the tiny serving size upon which the numbers are based. Look a little closer and you'll see that one popular butterlike spray contains 20 calories and 2 grams of fat per teaspoon, which is comparable to a low-fat spread. As for what you're actually spraying onto your food, well, let's just say you'll probably have no trouble believing it's not butter! Frankly, I can't see any advantage to spraying minute amounts of soybean oil, lecithin, xanthan gum, and yellow food coloring onto your food. It's not necessary to eliminate all fat from your diet. Brush on a small amount of real butter or olive oil and stop worrying about it.

EGGS

The dairy case also contains many items that have nothing to do with cows, such as eggs. For those who consume animal products, eggs are an inexpensive, convenient, and versatile source of high-quality protein. In fact, eggs contain all the essential amino acids (protein building blocks) in near-perfect proportions, which means that egg protein can be used very efficiently by the body.

The only thing you used to have to decide about your eggs was how big you wanted them. But here again, your options have exploded. Should you buy natural, organic, free-range, cage-free, pastured, or omega-3 fortified eggs? It depends on whether you're concerned with your own health, the health of the planet, the welfare of the egg layers, or all three. Here is a brief guide to what the various labels do (and don't) mean.

OMEGA-3 FORTIFIED—You get a little nutritional bonus from omega-3 fortified eggs. Omega-3 fatty acids are important to your immune function, brain, and heart health, and—as we repeatedly hear—most of us don't get nearly enough of them. Because they are always looking out for your needs (or at least your desires), manufacturers have come up with products to help fill the gap. To increase the omega-3 content of the eggs, the farmers put extra omega-3 in the chicken feed and the chickens do the rest. Omega-3 fortified eggs are not necessarily organic.

ORGANIC—Organic eggs come from chickens that are fed an organic, all-vegetarian diet that is free of antibiotics and pesticides. Pesticide residues are not generally found in eggs so paying more for organic eggs won't necessarily reduce your exposure to pesticides. It will, however, help keep the soil and water cleaner. Organic layers are not kept in cages and must have access to the outdoors, but if animal welfare is your main concern, you should know that organic eggs, along with eggs labeled "free-range," may come from chickens with extremely limited access to the outdoors. "Cage-free" layers typically do not have *any* access to the outdoors.

THE QUICK AND DIRTY SECRET

Organic eggs aren't necessarily any more nutritious or humanely produced than conventional eggs. Eggs from pastured hens are usually both.

PASTURED—If you like the idea of your chickens clucking happily around a roomy farmyard, nibbling green shoots and the occasional fat grub, eggs labeled "pastured" may come closer to your ideal, although this term is not strictly defined or regulated by any organization. Eggs from pastured chickens may or may not be organic, but because the chickens are allowed to forage for green plants and insects, their eggs are usually somewhat higher in beta-carotene, vitamin D, E, and omega-3 fatty acids. All of these particular nutrients, by the way, are found in the yolks. A chicken's diet doesn't really affect the egg whites, which are primarily protein.

Your Shopping Game Plan for Eggs

Eggs are an affordable source of high-quality protein. They're also versatile and quick to prepare. Eggs are rich in cholesterol, of course, and we used to worry that eating foods that contained cholesterol would cause high cholesterol levels. However, research shows that most healthy adults can eat a dozen or so eggs a week without adverse effects on their cholesterol levels or an increased risk of disease. Because fresh eggs will keep for several weeks in the refrigerator, I always keep a dozen on hand, even if I don't have a specific plan for them.

JUICE

Finally, although they have nothing to do with cows, fruit juices are typically found in the dairy section. A half cup of fruit juice technically counts as a serving of fruit but I consider processed fruit juice to be a distant second to fresh fruit, nutritionally. Processed fruit juice contains all of the sugar, some of the vitamins, and almost none of the fiber of fresh, whole fruit. As for those new fruit and vegetable juice blends that promise a serving of vegetables in every glass, any vegetables they may contain are vegetables in name only—not in terms of their nutritional value.

Frankly, I'd rather you skip the juice and eat another piece of fruit instead. (Or, at the very least, juice the fruit yourself right before you drink it.) I suggest limiting your juice intake to one serving a day and keep in mind that a serving is just one half cup. You'll get the most nutritional benefit from citrus, pomegranate, or grape juice and the least from apple juice. Diluting juice with spring water or sparkling water makes it more refreshing and (ounce for ounce) lower in sugar.

Special Note to Parents Fruit juice is not a good source of nutrition for your kids. It's a good source of sugar—natural sugars, but sugars all the same. You'll be doing your kids a huge favor by having them *eat* fruit and *drink* water.

If you're going to drink fruit juice, limit it to one serving per day. Citrus, pomegranate, and grape juice are the most nutritious choices.

THE MEAT DEPARTMENT

If you don't eat meat, you can skip this section. If you do, your first big decision might be whether to buy beef, chicken, or pork.

White Meat or Red Meat?

I'm always a little confused when I hear people claim that "white" meat, such as chicken and turkey, is better for you than "red" meat, such as beef and pork. Red meat contains up to twice as much iron, zinc, and vitamin B12 as poultry. White meat is not necessarily lower in fat, either. There are cuts of beef and pork that are just as lean as a boneless, skinless chicken breast. And, by the same token, there are cuts of chicken and turkey that have just as much fat as a well-marbled steak. Beef and pork also tend to contain a higher percentage of heart-healthy monounsaturated fats than turkey or chicken. So if you've been avoiding red meat on nutritional grounds, it may be time to rethink your boycott. Red and white meat can both be healthy choices. Whatever type of meat you buy, lean, well-trimmed cuts offer more protein and contain fewer calories per serving. Avoid things that have been "prebasted" or injected with salt or sugar solutions. Meat should contain meat and nothing else.

Best Choices in the Meat Department

Beef: tenderloin, strip steak, top sirloin, T-bone, flank steak, London broil

Bison: all

Lamb: loin chops, leg of lamb

Pork: tenderloin, loin roast

Poultry: skinless breast

Budget friendly: ground beef, bison, chicken, or turkey (90 percent lean), chuck roast (beef), skinless thighs (chicken)

How to Understand Meat Labels

Looking beyond the nutrition facts label, a lot of the terms you'll see on meat packages these days promise (or at least imply) something about how and where the animals were raised. Here's a quick guide to what some of these labels do (and don't) mean and how they affect the nutritional quality of the meat.

GRASS-FED/GRASS-FINISHED—With the adoption of new labeling regulations in 2010, these two terms now are equivalent. All cattle are typically raised on an open pasture for the first part of their lives; most are, and then fattened on grain before they are slaughtered. "Grass-fed" or "grass-finished" means that the cattle remain on pasture throughout their entire lives. In general, the beef is leaner, and a smaller proportion of the fat is saturated. Grass-fed beef may also be higher in vitamins A, E, and omega-3 fatty acids, although it is still not a significant source of these nutrients.

FREE-RANGE/CAGE-FREE—Usually applied to poultry and sometimes to pork, free-range means that the animals have access to the outdoors. However, free-range animals may still spend all or the majority of the time indoors and "outdoors" may mean a dirt yard or concrete slab. In terms of animal welfare, "free-range" may not mean a whole lot. And because these terms imply nothing about what the animals are fed, they don't have any meaning in terms of the nutritional quality of the meat.

PASTURED—This term is not regulated in the United States but it implies that the animals live on farms, not factories, and that they graze on an open pasture for a substantial part of their sustenance. Their diet may be supplemented by other feed. Pastured meats are generally the most animal- and environmentally friendly choices. They also offer some nutritional advantages. The meat may be leaner and have higher levels of vitamins A, E, and omega-3 fatty acids than conventionally raised meat.

KOSHER—Kosher refers mostly to how the animals are handled during and after they are slaughtered. Kosher meat is prepared under the supervision of a rabbi, according to traditional Jewish dietary laws. Nutritionally, the biggest difference is that kosher chicken is prepared with salt and may be higher in sodium.

HUMANELY RAISED—This term suggests that animals are raised and slaughtered using practices that preserve their quality of life and prevent undue physical or emotional stress. Although it is a self-regulated term, humanely raised animals are usually raised with access to a pasture and without the use of antibiotics or hormones.

ORGANIC—Certified organic meat comes from animals who are fed only organic food, which reduces the chemical burden on the environment. It also means that the meat should be free of pesticide residues—but meat is not a significant source of pesticide exposure. Organic meat is also produced without the use of antibiotics or growth hormones—and the implications of that go well beyond what is—or isn't—in the meat.

Meat from grass-fed or pastured animals is likely to be leaner and somewhat higher in certain nutrients than other meat.

What about Antibiotics in Meat?

The use of antibiotics in our livestock is a big problem for all of us, no matter what kind of meat we buy or even if we choose not to eat meat at all. As with people, antibiotics are used to treat sick animals. But in the United States, most livestock are also given low doses of antibiotics throughout their entire lives—sort of the way many people take vitamins. Putting antibiotics in the feed helps make the animals grow bigger, faster.

Growing more animals bigger and faster increases profits and, to some extent, keeps costs at the grocery store down. So what's the problem? The problem is that antibiotics are *not* vitamins. They are drugs that we depend on to fight infections that would otherwise kill millions of people every year. The way we are using antibiotics in livestock—constantly and in low doses—is the most efficient way to breed harmful bacteria that are resistant to those antibiotics.

Restricting the use of antibiotics in livestock would greatly reduce the dangers of antibiotic-resistant bacteria, but legislation has met with stiff resistance from the meat-growing industry. In the meantime, buying meat produced without antibiotics sends a message that consumers are willing to pay more for meat produced without antibiotics. Also, it helps support the farmers who opt out of the conventional system, and that reduces antibiotic use. Cutting back on antibiotic use in agriculture will help maintain the potency and viability of antibiotics to treat serious, life-threatening diseases in humans *and* animals.

Should You Buy Hormone-free Meat?

Hormones are not used in poultry or pork products. So, paying extra for hormone-free eggs or bacon is like paying extra for fat-free broccoli. But don't feel too bad if you fall for that one—lots of us did. They do, however, give hormones to cows—both dairy cows and the kind that are raised for meat. A variety of hormones—both natural and synthetic—are used to increase milk production and to make cows grow to their slaughter weight faster.

Environmentalists are worried that a lot of those hormones will end up in the cow's manure and make their way into streams and rivers, affecting fish, frogs, and other sensitive fauna. There are also fears that hormone residues in meat could affect the humans who consume them more directly, possibly affecting the age at which boys and girls reach puberty or increasing the risk of cancer.

Scientists point out that the level of hormones in meat is miniscule compared to the amount produced by our own bodies—and there's no solid evidence that these hormones have any effect on human health. Also, keep in mind that, though organic meat is raised without added hormones, it is not necessarily hormone-free. Cows produce their own hormones, after all. In fact, an untreated bull would have much higher levels of natural testosterone than a castrated steer that is receiving hormone replacement therapy.

Public health agencies are split on the issue. The European Union, for example, has outlawed the use of hormones in cattle and banned beef imports from the United States due to their concerns. The U.S. FDA, on the other hand, insists that the use of hormones in beef and dairy cattle poses no threat to human welfare and that meat and milk from cows given hormones is identical to meat and milk produced without hormones. If you want meat raised without hormones in the United States, you'll want to buy certified organic.

Beef produced without hormones isn't more nutritious than regular meat, nor is it likely to be hormone-free. But because giving cattle hormones may ultimately have harmful effects on the environment and consumers, I think it's worth the money. (Don't worry about looking for hormone-free pork or poultry products as these animals aren't given hormones in the first place.)

Cold Cuts and Cured Meats

Cured meats, including ham, bacon, hot dogs, bologna, salami, and other hard sausages tend to be high in sodium and fat. Worse, they usually contain nitrates and nitrites. These compounds have been linked to cancer in both lab animals and humans. If you only eat these types of foods occasionally, I don't think you need to be concerned about this. But these aren't foods you want to be eating in large quantities or on a regular basis.

Developing fetuses and small children seem to be the most vulnerable to the carcinogenic effects of nitrites. Pregnant women and small children should avoid cured meats altogether.

Nitrite-free hot dogs, boloney, and ham are also an option—although be forewarned that they won't be that bright pink color that you're used to. Nitrites are what turn ham, hot dogs, and cold cuts pink. Nitrite-free versions taste exactly the same but they're usually tan or brown.

Deli meats such as sliced turkey breast, chicken, or roast beef are generally nitrite free. They're also low in fat. They can be saltier than fresh meats, however, so if sodium is a concern, look for the reduced-sodium variety.

Your Shopping Game Plan for Meat

Calculate servings. Figure how many servings you'll need based on the number of people in your household and the number of meals at which you'll be serving meat between now and your next shopping trip. Keep in mind that meat doesn't have to be a daily event. With seafood and vegetarian meals also in your repertoire and the occasional meal out, you may only end up serving meat once or twice a week.

Estimate portions. Four ounces of uncooked, boneless meat will yield approximately three ounces of cooked meat—and that's the standard serving size on which most dietary recommendations are based. However, the portions commonly served in restaurants—and many homes—are usually about twice that big. A one-pound (16-ounce) flank steak or pork tenderloin, for example, will yield four small servings or two large ones. For cuts that include bones, expect to get two to three small servings or one large serving per pound of uncooked meat. A three-pound whole chicken, for example, will yield six small servings or three large ones.

Stretch your budget. You can save money by stocking your freezer when there are specials. Just be sure the meat has not previously been frozen and don't stock more than you'll eat within two to three months.

Be your own deli. If you are roasting a chicken or roast beef for dinner, plan to use the leftovers for sandwiches and salads and skip the deli.

Plan meals on the fly. As you make your selections, think about how you'll serve them and what you might need for those meals or recipes. For example, that ground bison would make a great pot of chili. If you're low on beans or chili powder, add those to your list. (See my recipe for Chili con Cocoa on page 220.)

THE FISH COUNTER

Health experts recommend eating at least two servings of fish a week for better health. And although fish consumption is up somewhat, we're still falling short of the goal, eating closer to one serving a week on average. We can do better! Here are some of the factors to consider when choosing fish, along with guidelines to help you zero in on the best choices.

OMEGA-3 FATS—One big reason we're all encouraged to eat more fish is that it can be a good source of omega-3 fatty acids. These important fats support a healthy immune system and help keep your brain and cardiovascular system healthy. Although all fish and shellfish are generally nutritious, certain fish are particularly rich in omega-3 fatty acids. As a rule, fish with oilier, stronger-tasting meat are higher in omega-3 fats. The following fish are high in omega-3 fats:

Salmon
Herring
Mackerel
Sardines
Anchovies
Sablefish (aka black cod)
Bluefin tuna (albacore and yellowfin are much lower in
    Omega-3)
Whitefish
Caviar
Rainbow trout

THE QUICK AND DIRTY SECRET

Of the recommended two servings of fish a week, try to make at least one of them a type that's high in omega-3s.

MERCURY—Virtually all fish contain mercury. But this is not a reason to avoid seafood. There have been countless studies connecting fish eating to greater health and longevity, and mercury poisoning is rare, even in people who eat a lot of fish. That would suggest that the benefits of eating fish outweigh the risks—with one exception. Exposure to mercury—which can affect the development of the nervous system—is most dangerous to fetuses and small children. Pregnant and nursing women and small children avoid fish known to be high in mercury. People who eat fish more than twice a week might want to follow the same precautions. Everyone else can relax. The following fish are high in mercury:

> Shark
> Swordfish
> King mackerel
> Tilefish
> Albacore ("white") tuna

THE QUICK AND DIRTY SECRET

Pregnant women, small children, and those who eat fish more than twice a week should watch out for fish that are high in mercury.

PCBs—Although PCBs were banned years ago, they persist in the environment, tending to accumulate in riverbeds and shallow sea beds. From here they make their way into fish and, ultimately, into us. PCBs are suspected carcinogens and repeated exposure may also cause neurological or other problems, especially in babies and young children.

As with mercury, it's important to put this into perspective. It would appear that the benefits of eating fish outweigh the health risks from contaminants. Nonetheless, as with fish containing high levels of mercury, it makes sense to limit your consumption of those fish known to be particularly high in PCB residues. The following fish are high in PCBs:

Bluefish
Striped bass (wild)
Croaker
Sturgeon
Flounder
Rockfish
Rainbow trout (farmed)

SUSTAINABILITY—Finally, now that we're all trying to eat more fish, there are concerns that growing demand is quickly depleting wild populations. At the same time, overcrowded fish farms are polluting the environment. These factors may not affect the nutritional quality of the fish itself but, as with hormones and antibiotics in livestock, supporting sustainable fishing practices makes sense when you consider the long-term view. Because fish is so good for us, we want to be sure we don't run out of it. We also don't want to destroy the environment in the process.

Some of the fish that are a particular concern right now include:

Chilean sea bass
Cobie
Marlin
Monkfish
Grouper
Orange roughy
Shark
Swordfish
Tilefish
Tuna, (bluefin, bigeye, yellowfin)

How to Keep Track

Frankly, it's a lot to keep track of. No wonder we're tempted to skip the fish counter entirely. However, there are a couple of tools that make it simple to make the best choices. You can download and print out a pocket-sized Seafood Selector and Sushi Guide from the Environmental Defense Fund at www.edf.org. There are also a number of

Smartphone applications, such as Seafood Watch from the Monterey Bay Aquarium.

Frozen and Canned Fish

If fresh fish is expensive or the selection is limited (or you find the prospect of selecting or cooking fresh fish intimidating), frozen and canned fish can be good alternatives. Canned fish like sardines, anchovies, and salmon offer a nutritional bonus. In addition to being high in omega-3 fatty acids, they are also high in calcium. Most canned fish is fairly high in sodium, however. If you're trying to keep your sodium down, you'll want to budget your sodium allowance and your canned fish intake accordingly. With frozen fish, steer clear of breaded and battered options.

Best Choices for Fish

Taking all of the previous issues into consideration, the fish below are good choices all around.

TYPE	BEST CHOICES	BUDGET-FRIENDLY
fresh	Arctic char wild salmon sablefish (black cod) oysters (farmed)	cod haddock
frozen	wild salmon shrimp	cod haddock
canned	wild Alaska pink salmon Alaskan sockeye sardines anchovies	chunk light tuna

Your Shopping Game Plan for Fish

Estimate Portions A small serving of fish is about four ounces of uncooked fish. A larger serving, such as the size served in most restaurants, is closer to eight ounces uncooked. So if you're buying salmon to cook for six people, a 24-ounce fillet will give you six small servings or three large ones. If you're buying a whole fish, plan on double the weight per serving. Your goal is to have at least two small servings (or one large serving) of fish every week. That doesn't mean you necessarily have to buy and cook fish every week. Meals you eat in restaurants count as well—as does the tuna sandwich you take for lunch.

Keep It Fresh Fish does not keep well, so plan to cook (or freeze) fresh fish the day you buy it. Cool storage is also crucial, so ask the grocer to give you a bag of ice to carry the fish home in and store it in the fridge, ice and all, until it's time to cook.

Have A Backup Plan Canned or frozen fish are good budget-friendly options to keep on hand for last-minute meals. Although canned fish will keep indefinitely, frozen fish should be consumed within two or three months.

Plan Meals On The Fly If a beautiful piece of fish catches your eye for dinner tonight, think about what you might like to serve with it and add those items to your list. Grilled salmon goes particularly well with Asian-style Broccoli Salad, for example (see my recipe on page 204). So well, in fact, that once you see that wild-caught salmon on special, you'll probably want to circle back to the produce section and grab some broccoli, if you didn't already pick some up. And if you're running low on seasoned rice vinegar, be sure to add that to your list, as well.

We've now pretty much completed our circuit around the edges of the store. Hopefully, your cart is pretty full by now. But there are still a few things that you'll probably need to round out your meals and menus. It's time to head into the interior aisles.

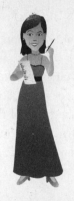

CHAPTER TWO

Stocking the Pantry

IN THIS CHAPTER, we'll take a look at various foods I think of as "pantry staples"—grains, beans, oils, nuts, canned vegetables, and so on. I'll help you pick out the best choices and tell you what to avoid in each category. Like the foods around the perimeter of the store, most of these pantry staples are single-ingredient items, such as rice or olive oil. I've also included bread, pastas, and cereal in this chapter, even though they usually have slightly longer ingredient lists.

GRAINS

One of the reasons that grains have become such a central part of the human diet is that they have a long shelf life. Unlike meat, dairy, and fresh produce, grains pack a whole lot of food energy (also known as calories) into a small, lightweight package that can be stored indefinitely without refrigeration or other preservation. If you've got some dirt and a water supply, your last handful of grain can be used to create the next season's food supply. You can see why they caught on.

Although grains are portable and nonperishable, they're not really edible in their raw state. You can boil, steam, or sprout whole grains and eat them that way. Or you can mill the grains into flour and use it to make bread, tortillas, or pasta. Either way, it's considered a whole-grain food if all of the parts of the grain are included—the nutrient-rich germ, the starchy endosperm, and the fibrous bran. When the bran and germ have been removed, as in white flour, it's said to be a refined grain.

The Advantages of Whole-grain Foods

Keeping the germ makes whole-grain foods somewhat higher in certain vitamins and minerals. But the primary nutritional advantage of whole grains is that the fiber from the bran slows down the speed at which the starches in the endosperm are converted into blood sugar. Said another way, whole-grain foods have a lower glycemic load, and when you're talking about glycemic load, lower is generally better. Foods with a high glycemic load tend to make your blood sugar and insulin spike, which increases your risk of diabetes and heart disease and can potentially lead to weight gain, as well. In fact, diets high in refined grains (which have a high glycemic load) have been linked to heart disease, type 2 diabetes, cancer, and obesity. Choosing whole grains instead of refined grains reduces these risks. Even better, try to eat most of your whole grains as intact grains rather than flour.

The Difference Between Whole Grains and Intact Grains

The terminology used to describe grains can be a little confusing. Breads, cereals, pasta, and other foods can be labeled "whole grain" if they're made with whole grain *flour*. But obviously, once you've ground a kernel of wheat or rice into a pile of dust, it's not really "whole" anymore. To avoid confusion, I use the term "intact grains" to refer to grains that are still more or less in their original shape.

Most of the dietary guidelines you'll come across emphasize the importance of whole grains, but they rarely distinguish between intact whole grains and milled whole- grains, or flour. In fact, there are some important differences. Intact grains are digested and absorbed more slowly than milled grains, which is generally a plus. And although whole grain flour contains all the parts of the original grain, some nutrients are lost or degraded in the milling process. For these reasons, I consider intact whole grains a notch above foods made with whole-grain flour. And the more grain-based foods you eat, the more important the quality of those grains becomes.

THE QUICK AND DIRTY SECRET

Whole grains are good, whole intact grains are better, and refined grains should be consumed in limited quantities.

LET'S TAKE A CLOSER LOOK

Do You Need to Eat Grains?

The current dietary guidelines recommend that you get a minimum of three servings of whole grains every day, based on research showing that people whose diets are high in whole grains have lower rates of heart disease and diabetes compared with people whose diets are high in refined grains. It's pretty clear that replacing refined grains with whole grains is helpful. What's not as clear is whether those benefits come from eating more whole grains or from eating less refined grains. Some people argue that you'd be better off without any grains at all. Although I think it's possible to have a healthy diet that includes them, I agree that grains are not essential.

Rice

Of all the grains that are cooked and eaten whole, rice is probably the most familiar. But there are at least a dozen different types of rice to choose from at the grocery store, all with very different properties.

SHORT-GRAIN—Almost as wide as it is long, short-grain rice is very starchy and cooks up soft and sticky. It's used in things like sushi, paella, and risotto.

LONG-GRAIN—Because it contains less starch, long-grain rice is drier and more separate when cooked. It's often used in pilafs or dishes with a lot of sauce.

JASMINE AND BASMATI—Long-grain varieties that have been culti-vated to bring out distinctive flavor profiles. They often turn up in Indian and Asian food.

INSTANT OR CONVERTED—Partially cooked and then dehydrated to shorten cooking times.

All of these are available as white (refined) or brown (whole grain). Because it retains both the germ and the bran parts of the grain, brown rice is higher in magnesium and other minerals than white rice. It also has about four times more fiber. As a general rule, brown rice has a lower glycemic load than white rice, thanks to the extra fi-ber. But other factors come into play as well. Long-grain rice has a lower glycemic load than short-grain rice. Of all the long-grain rice, basmati seems to have the lowest glycemic load of all.

Best Choices for Rice

Lower glycemic load (for white rice): basmati
Higher in fiber and nutrients: brown rice

In addition to rice, you'll find several other types of grains, each with unique texture, taste, and nutritional profile. Adding some of these less common grains into the rotation is a great way to add variety to your diet. All of the following, with the exception of pearled barley, are whole grains. And all, with the exception of barley and bulgur, are gluten free. (See "Should You Go Gluten-free?" on page 53.) Although you can buy preseasoned mixes, they are often high in sodium. Plain, unadulterated grains offer the best value and are free of salt and other additives. I'll have tips in chapter 7 on how to make flavorful grain dishes.

Guide to Grains

AMARANTH—Small, golden grains that stick together when cooked, resembling polenta. It's high in protein, iron, and calcium but also higher in calories than many grains due to its higher fat content.

BULGUR—Whole wheat that's been steamed, dehydrated, and cracked into small pieces and rehydrated. It's higher in fiber and lower in calories than most grains.

BARLEY—Sold hulled or pearled, barley is a medium-sized grain that cooks into a light, slightly slippery, pastalike texture. Barley is a decent source of iron and fiber but one of the lowest in protein.

BUCKWHEAT (KASHA)—Dark-colored grains are hulled and cracked and (for kasha) toasted. Cooked grains are hearty and separate. It's lower in carbohydrates and calories than most grains.

MILLET—Small, light-colored grain. Cooked grains are mild-tasting and separate. Millet is in the middle of the pack in terms of protein, but lower in fiber than most whole grains.

OAT—Most familiar as a breakfast grain, oats are usually rolled into flakes or cracked (steel-cut). Flakes cook to a porridge consistency; steel-cut remain more separate. Oats are moderate in protein and fiber but a bit lower in carbohydrates than many grains.

POLENTA—Whole corn milled into coarse or fine grits. Can be cooked into a mush or stiffer consistency. Polenta is lower in calories and carbohydrates than many grains but also low in protein and fiber.

QUINOA—Small, light-colored grains that remain separate when cooked, with a nutty flavor. Quinoa is among the higher-protein grains but also on the higher end in terms of calories per serving.

TEFF—Very small, dark brown grain, cooks to a stiff mush. Teff is among the highest in protein but also relatively high in carbohydrates and calories. It is also a good source of iron and calcium.

WILD RICE—Dark brown grains have chewy sheath and tender interior; grains remain separate when cooked, resembling long-grain rice. Wild rice is low in calories and a good source of vitamin A, folic acid, and omega-3 fats.

If you're wondering where couscous is, surprise! It's actually not a grain at all. See the next section on pasta.

Best Choices in Grains

Higher in protein: teff, amaranth, quinoa
Higher in fiber: bulgur
Lower in carbohydrates and calories: buckwheat, bulgur, polenta, oats, wild rice
Higher in calcium and iron: amaranth, teff
Higher in omega-3: quinoa, wild rice

PASTA

Pasta is made by grinding grains (usually wheat) into flour, mixing it with liquid to create a dough, and rolling or squeezing it into an astonishing variety of shapes. The dough, which may be fresh or dried, is boiled before eating. Pasta has gotten a bad reputation as some sort of carbohydrate nightmare. But I'm not sure that reputation is entirely deserved. For example, a one cup serving of cooked pasta contains the same amount of carbs as does a cup of rice.

Couscous: Grain or Pasta?

Although many people categorize couscous as a grain, it is actually a pasta. It comes in two sizes—standard couscous is similar to the size and texture of bulgur wheat and Israeli couscous is the size of barley grains. Couscous may be made from whole grain or refined wheat flour.

Pasta may be made with white or whole-grain flour; the latter offers more fiber. The main benefit of the extra fiber in whole-grain pasta is that it slightly reduces the amount of digestible carbohydrate in each serving and slows down the speed at which the carbohydrates are converted into blood sugar. In other words, whole-grain pasta has a lower glycemic load. It's also quite a bit heavier and coarser than regular pasta.

There are some new products on the market (such as Barilla PLUS pasta) that offer some of the benefits of whole grain but have a texture and flavor that's similar to pasta made from white flour. In addition to wheat flour, these pastas include flour from peas, lentils, and other legumes, which add extra protein and fiber as well as "resistant starches," which are discussed on pages 52–53. As a result, they are somewhat lower in digestible carbohydrates and higher in protein than regular pasta. For those who avoid wheat or gluten (See "Should You Go Gluten-free?" on page 53), you can also find pasta made from rice, quinoa, and other alternative grains. Because the gluten in wheat is a big part of what gives pasta its characteristic texture, wheat-free pastas may take some getting used to. Most alternative pastas are also quite a bit lower in protein than wheat pasta.

> ## Best Choices in Pasta
>
> **Higher in protein:** pasta made with legume flour (such as Barilla PLUS), egg noodles
> **Higher in fiber:** whole wheat
> **Lower in carbohydrates:** egg, whole wheat
> **Lower in calories:** quinoa

What Are Resistant Starches?

Some foods contain a type of starch that is resistant to digestive enzymes. Instead of being broken down into sugar molecules and absorbed into the bloodstream, resistant starches act more like fiber, passing through the system undigested. Resistant starches are found naturally in dried beans, as well as underripe bananas and mangos. And when you cook starchy foods such as potatoes, rice, and pasta, some of the regular starches are converted to resistant starches as the food cools. (So, for example, a cold pasta or potato salad will contain a bit more resistant starch than freshly cooked pasta or a baked potato.)

Adding resistant starches to your diet offers a number of potential benefits:

IMPROVED BOWEL FUNCTION—As with fiber, adding resistant starch to your diet can improve regularity and bowel function. Some people find that when they increase their fiber intake, especially if they do it suddenly, they have bloating, gas pains, and other effects usually lumped together under the heading of "gastrointestinal distress." One nice thing about resistant starch is that it doesn't have this unwelcome side effect.

APPETITE CONTROL—Another fiberlike benefit of resistant starch is that it appears to help with appetite control, enabling you to feel fuller for longer, even when you are eating fewer calories.

BLOOD-SUGAR REGULATION—When you include resistant starches in a meal, it slows down the absorption of sugars from other foods. That means that you get a more gradual rise and fall in blood-sugar levels after eating. That's particularly helpful for diabetics, who need to keep their blood-sugar levels steady. But the blood-sugar roller coaster isn't a ride you want to be on, even if you're not diabetic.

CALORIE REDUCTION—Foods containing a lot of resistant starches are somewhat lower in calories than other carbohydrates because at least some of the food energy stays locked up in the resistant starch and doesn't get digested and absorbed.

You get the benefits of resistant starches naturally by including more legumes in your diet. Manufacturers sometimes add legume flour or high amylase corn starch (a resistant starch extracted from corn) to high-carbohydrate foods such as pasta, bread, and cereal to make them lower in calories and carbohydrates. Resistant starches are often used in foods marketed to diabetics and low-carb dieters.

LET'S TAKE A CLOSER LOOK

Should You Go Gluten-free?

Gluten is a protein found in wheat and certain other cereal grains, including rye and barley. For people with celiac disease, this protein triggers an immune reaction that, if left untreated, can cause permanent damage to the lining of the small intestine. Untreated celiac disease also can lead to serious nutritional deficiencies because the damaged intestines are not able to absorb important nutrients. Celiac is not the same as a wheat allergy or gluten intolerance, although these can cause similar symptoms. And the solution for all three conditions is the same: a gluten-free diet will relieve symptoms and, in the case of celiac disease, prevent permanent damage to the bowel lining.

The benefits of a gluten-free diet for people with celiac disease, wheat allergies, or gluten intolerance are fairly obvious. But gluten-free products are also developing some cachet with people who don't have these problems. I suspect that some people aren't even sure what gluten is but when you see "gluten-free" on a package, it suggests that gluten is something to be avoided.

The truth is that many people—even most people—tolerate gluten just fine. Yet you often hear stories from people who say that removing gluten from their diets cured them of their long-standing sinusitis, joint pain, irritable bowel, acne, or fatigue. Whether it was truly the gluten that was causing these symptoms is hard to say. But if you feel better when you cut out gluten, you're not missing anything nutritionally.

BREADS

Although it's sometimes referred to as the staff of life, bread is not actually essential to a healthy diet. Nonetheless, it has its place. For one thing, it keeps your hands tidy when you eat sandwiches. But the more bread you eat, the more important it is to choose bread made with whole grains rather than refined white flour.

Finding the whole-grain bread among the dozens of options on the shelves isn't as simple as it sounds. You can't go by the color: Manufacturers sometimes add molasses or even food coloring to mimic the darker color of whole grains. They use virtuous-sounding terms like "stone-ground," "100 percent wheat," "multigrain," or "made with whole grains" to describe their products. They might even add ingredients that create a dense, chewy texture. None of these things are a reliable indicator of whole grains.

A "multigrain" bread, for example, could be made out of several types of *refined* grains. Or, more likely, it's made with lots of refined white flour and small amounts of other whole grains. Your best bet is to ignore most of the words on the package and zero in on the ingredient list. Look specifically for the word "whole" right before the name of the grain, as in "whole wheat" or "whole oats." Keep in mind that the ingredients listed first are the ones that make up the bulk of the product. As a general rule, whole-grain bread should have at least three grams of fiber per serving. Whole-grain tortillas, pita, rolls, buns, and English muffins are all interchangeable with whole-grain breads (and the same guidelines apply).

THE QUICK AND DIRTY SECRET

Look for breads that contain at least 3 grams of fiber per serving.

What Is Sprouted-grain Bread?

Are breads made from sprouted grains more nutritious? Sprouting a seed (or grain) can increase its protein and vitamin content—and fresh sprouts can be a nutritious addition to any diet. However, once these sprouted grains have been milled, dried, and baked into breads and other products, the nutritional advantages don't add up to much. Nutritionally speaking, sprouted-grain breads are comparable to other whole-grain breads.

Are There Health Benefits to Sourdough?

Sourdough bread is leavened with a mixture of yeast and lactobacillus bacteria, which impart the characteristic sourdough "tang." Consuming foods containing live and active cultures of these friendly bacteria can be beneficial (See "Yogurt and Other Friends with Benefits," page 24). Unfortunately, the organisms are destroyed at baking temperatures, so you won't get those particular benefits from sourdough bread. Sourdough does offer one potential advantage, however. It is higher in resistant starch than bread made with regular yeast. (See "What Are Resistant Starches?", page 52.) The end result is that sourdough bread doesn't create as quick an increase in blood sugar as regular bread does. You can maximize this effect by choosing whole-grain sourdough breads.

What Is White Whole-wheat Bread?

"White whole-wheat bread" seems too good to be true, but isn't. In this case, "white" refers to the variety of wheat ("red" is the more typical type). Whole-grain bread made from white wheat is soft and light—it looks and feels more like white bread than whole wheat. Nevertheless, 100 percent white whole-wheat bread counts as a whole-grain bread.

What about Low-caloric Bread?

You'll also find "light breads" that are promoted as being lower in calories or carbohydrates. Some of these are simply regular bread sliced thinner (ta-daa!). But others cut carbohydrates by replacing some of the flour with protein powder, fiber, or resistant starch. (See "What Are Resistant Starches?" on page 52.) These ingredients aren't unhealthy but some people find that they make bread a little tough, dry, or odd-tasting. (Toasting the bread sometimes helps.) Most give you two slices for the same amount of calories and carbohydrates as one slice of regular bread. If you're in the market for a low-carbohydrate bread, look for one that provides at least 3 grams of fiber per serving

CEREAL

Nowhere is the folly and excess of the processed foods industry more apparent than in the cereal aisle. You'll find scores of brightly colored boxes filled with flakes, nuggets, clusters, squares, and Os, fortified with basic vitamins and minerals as well as more exotic nutrients, all designed to get our (or the kids') day off to a healthy start. To compete for their share of this extremely profitable market, cereal makers just keep piling on the exotic ingredients (grape-seed extract! prebiotics! omega-3s!) and the health claims (lowers cholesterol! promotes weight loss! builds strong bones!). Don't be overly impressed.

All of these nutrients and benefits are available from less-processed and less expensive foods.

My complaint with most breakfast cereals—even the ones that are designed to appeal to the health-conscious consumer—is that they are shockingly high in added sugar. Your highest priority with ready-to-eat cereal is to avoid excessive amounts of sugar. Your second priority is to choose cereals that provide a decent amount of fiber. Everything else is a bonus. If the cereal is loaded with sugar, it largely cancels out the benefit of that grape-seed extract.

Hot Cereals

Hot cereals like oatmeal, steel-cut oats, or multigrain porridge are great whole grain options—but the Rule of Five generally rules out the flavored varieties, which are loaded with sugar. In terms of vitamins, minerals, and fiber, the differences between regular and quick-cooking or instant oats are fairly minimal. Perhaps the biggest difference is that the carbohydrates in instant oats are more quickly absorbed and converted into blood sugar. That is to say, they have a slightly higher glycemic load. If you're hooked on the add-boiling-water-and-stir convenience of instant oatmeal, it's still a much better choice than cereals with added sugar. But in chapter 4, I have a tip on how to make regular oats just as quick and convenient as instant.

The Rule of Five

When shopping for cereal, check the Nutrition Facts label, using my Rule of Five as a guide. Ideally, cereal should have less than 5 grams of sugar and 5 grams or more of fiber per serving. The Rule of Five is not set in stone. If a cereal is very low in sugar, it's okay if it's also a little lower in fiber. For example, oatmeal has only 4 grams of fiber per serving but 0 grams of sugar. On the other hand, cereals that contain dried fruit may be higher in sugar. Just be sure that most of the sugar is, indeed, coming from fruit and not from added sugars. (If sugar or corn syrup are among the first few ingredients in the list, pass on it).

Look for cereal with less than 5 grams of sugar and 5 grams or more of fiber per serving.

FLOUR

The various flours differ in their nutritional qualities but also in their uses and characteristics: You may wish to keep a couple of different kinds on hand. Substituting whole-grain flour for white flour in recipes can improve the food's nutritional value but it will also dramatically change the flavor, texture, and other properties of baked goods, including baking or rising times. For best results, start by substituting a small portion of the flour—perhaps a quarter of what's called for—and see how you like the results before increasing it further. Even better, look for recipes that are specifically developed for whole-grain or other alternative flours.

The more you do your own cooking, of course, the more control you have over what goes into your food! Here's a quick guide to the different types of flour you might come across.

ORGANIC—Whether white or whole grain, organic flour is made from grains that are grown without synthetic herbicides or pesticides and will be free of residues from these chemicals. Choosing organic products also helps reduce the use of agricultural chemicals, which benefits the environment.

ALL-PURPOSE WHITE FLOUR—Made from wheat, with the bran and germ removed. Baked goods made from white flour are lighter in texture and color but lower in fiber than those made from whole grains. All-purpose flour may be bleached or unbleached, but the two are nutritionally equivalent.

BREAD FLOUR—Higher in protein, which helps bread rise better but can make other baked goods, such as pancakes or muffins, somewhat tough.

WHOLE WHEAT FLOUR—Retains the germ and bran and is higher in fiber than white flour. Substituting whole wheat flour for white flour in recipes will make baked goods more nutritious but also heavier and coarser. Breads made with whole-wheat flour take longer to rise and usually will not rise as high.

WHITE WHOLE-WHEAT FLOUR—A whole-grain flour with all of the nutritional advantages of regular whole-wheat flour. However, it's made from a different strain of wheat that is much lighter in color and texture. When modifying recipes, white whole-wheat makes a much better substitute for white bread flour than traditional whole-wheat flour does.

WHOLE-WHEAT PASTRY FLOUR—Similar in color and flavor to traditional whole-wheat flour but lower in protein. It's best for baked goods made without yeast, such as muffins, cakes, quick breads, and scones. When modifying recipes, whole-wheat pastry flour makes a better substitute for all-purpose flour than traditional whole-wheat flour does.

GLUTEN FLOUR—A high-protein wheat flour that can be used in whole-grain bread recipes to strengthen the dough and enhance rising.

KAMUT AND SPELT FLOUR—Whole-grain flours that can be used in place of whole-wheat flour. Both grains are closely related to wheat—think of them as "heirloom" varieties of today's standard wheat. They are nutritionally similar to regular whole-wheat flour.

NONWHEAT FLOUR—Virtually any grain can be milled into flour. You'll find many of the grains listed on page 50 also come as flour, including amaranth, buckwheat, millet, oat, and rice. None of these flours have any gluten, which means that they do not make good substitutes for wheat flour in baked goods that depend on gluten for their structure and texture (which is almost all of them). When using these flours, your best bet is to use recipes developed specifically for them.

HI-MAIZE—A flour replacement made from modified cornstarch. Because it's high in resistant starch, it's much lower in carbohydrates and calories than regular flour. It can be used to replace some (10 to 25 percent) of the white flour in recipes, reducing the amount of digestible carbohydrates and calories in your baked goods. (See "What Are Resistant Starches?" page 52.)

SWEETENERS

Sweeteners rank at the lower end of the nutrition spectrum, but you don't have to avoid them completely.

Sugar

I'm sure you've heard enough about how bad refined sugar is for your health to think twice before putting that bag of white sugar into your grocery cart. But what about evaporated cane juice or raw sugar? Are these "natural" sugars really better for you than refined white sugar? Or, at the very least, are they a little less bad for you? The idea of calling white sugar "refined" and raw sugar "natural" is a little silly. All of these sugars are natural in the sense that they all come from plants. And all of these sugars are refined. They've all been extracted from cane or beet and dried into a crystalline form. The ones that we call "natural" are just a little bit less refined. Advertisers try to make it sound as if these less-refined sugars are also more nutritious than regular white sugar. They claim that they retain more of the nutrients from the original plant. And, technically, that may be true. But sugarcane doesn't have many nutrients to start out with. Any traces that remain in raw sugar are so trivial, they can barely be measured.

Nutritionally speaking, there really is no meaningful difference between any of these kinds of sugar. Although some are definitely less processed, they all provide the same number of calories, and when it comes to digestion and metabolism, your body cannot tell the difference. More to the point, all concentrated sugars, whether natural or not, are foods that should be consumed in moderation with a capital M.

THE QUICK AND DIRTY SECRET

Nutritionally speaking, evaporated cane juice crystals and raw sugar are no better for you than regular white sugar.

The Different Types of Sugar

Here's a guide to the types of sugar commonly found in most grocery stores.

REFINED WHITE SUGAR—Can be produced from either sugarcane or sugar beets, but by the time it has been refined to a white crystal, the two are chemically identical—virtually pure sucrose.

BROWN SUGAR—Refined white sugar with some coloring and flavoring added back into it.

EVAPORATED CANE JUICE—Made from sugarcane (never sugar beets), it's slightly less refined and so it retains a bit more color and flavor from the sugar cane. The tan-colored crystals have a slight caramel or molasses aroma. If the crystals are large and coarse, it's also known as demerara sugar.

TURBINADO OR "RAW" SUGAR—Dehydrated cane juice that retains a bit more of the natural "impurities," so it's even a little darker and the molasses aroma and flavor is a bit more pronounced.

ORGANIC CANE SUGAR—From sugarcane that's grown without synthetic herbicides or pesticides. It may be lightly refined or almost pure white. Not only will the sugar itself be free of residues from these chemicals, but choosing organic products also reduces the overall pesticide load on the environment.

Best Choices in Sugar

Least refined: raw sugar
Best substitute for white sugar: evaporated cane juice
Most eco-friendly: organic

Should You Eliminate Sugar from Your Diet?

Some people will tell you that in order to be healthy, you must completely eliminate sugar from your diet. If you're inclined to do this, you have my full support, as well as my respect. Obviously, you won't be missing out on a thing, nutritionally. Sugar is a nutritional zero. In fact, when consumed in excess, it's worse than zero; it can have very negative effects. The amount of sugar we are consuming these days—about a half cup per day, on average—is clearly to blame for many of our fastest growing health problems, such as obesity, diabetes, and heart disease. I don't want to pull any punches here: If your diet is high in sugar (and you're probably eating more than you realize), cutting back on sugar is probably *the most important thing* you can do to improve your diet and your health. However, I think a zero-tolerance policy may be unnecessarily extreme. Though sugar provides no nutritional benefits, it makes life a little bit sweeter. Small amounts (and I do mean small) are not going to derail an otherwise healthy diet. We'll talk more about this as we go through the book, but the goal is to reduce that one-half cup to just a couple of tablespoons or so of sugar per day. At that point, however, you can stop worrying about it!

Liquid Sweeteners

Compared with sugar, liquid sweeteners like honey and maple syrup are a step closer to nature and marginally higher in certain nutrients—but this is not license to overindulge. Nutritionally, liquid sweeteners are in the same category as regular sugar: concentrated sources of sugar and calories. Liquid sweeteners can be used in place of sugar to sweeten cereal or beverages. In recipes, however, substitute with caution. Not only are there pronounced differences in flavor, but you will probably need to increase or decrease the amount to get the desired level of sweetness and may need to adjust the amount of other liquid ingredients.

AGAVE SYRUP—Higher in sugar and calories than the same amount of cane sugar but it tastes quite a bit sweeter, so you may be able to use less. Agave syrup causes a much smaller rise in blood sugar than other caloric sweeteners.

BROWN RICE SYRUP—Comparable to cane sugar in sweetness but higher in calories. It causes a somewhat smaller rise in blood sugar than other caloric sweeteners.

HONEY—Higher in calories than the same amount of cane sugar, but because it tastes a bit sweeter, you may be able to use less. It causes a somewhat smaller rise in blood sugar than other caloric sweeteners.

Fructose: Sweet or Sinister?

Certain sweeteners—such as agave nectar, brown rice syrup, and honey—have a higher proportion of fructose, a type of sugar that does not raise your blood sugar. Of all the liquid sweeteners, agave nectar is particularly high in fructose and, correspondingly, has a very minimal impact on blood sugar. However, there are some downsides: Large amounts of fructose can signal your body to store more fat. It can also raise your triglycerides, a type of blood fat that increases your risk of heart disease. The take-home message? All sweeteners should be consumed in moderation.

MAPLE SYRUP—Contains about the same amount of calories and sugar as cane sugar but tastes less sweet and causes a slightly smaller rise in blood sugar.

MOLASSES—Everything that is left behind when sugarcane is refined into white sugar. It contains small amounts of calcium, iron, and other minerals. Although it is higher in calories than the same amount of cane sugar, it tastes quite a bit less sweet and causes a slightly smaller rise in blood sugar.

Best Choices in Liquid Sugar

Most nutrients: molasses
Lowest in calories: maple syrup
Least effect on blood sugar: agave, honey

Sugar Substitutes

Zero-calorie sweeteners offer a way to enjoy sweets without the negative consequences of sugar. They add no calories to your diet. They have no effect on blood-sugar levels, which can be helpful for diabetics. And, of course, unlike sugar, artificial sweeteners don't cause tooth decay. But there's no such thing as a free lunch, and zero-calorie sweeteners have some downsides, as well. First, many people find their super-sweet taste and bitter, chemical aftertaste unpleasant. Secondly, using sugar substitutes to make cookies or other baked goods is almost always disappointing because real sugar is crucial to things like texture and browning.

LET'S TAKE A CLOSER LOOK

Are Artificial Sweeteners Safe?

Despite the fact that all of the artificial sweeteners have been approved for human consumption and are considered safe, some people are concerned that artificial sweeteners might be toxic or cause cancer. I don't actually worry too much about this—and not because I think our regulatory agencies flawlessly protect us from unsafe products. I don't worry about it because these products have been so heavily consumed for such a long time that if there were a connection between their use and brain cancer or something else, I think we would have seen something by now. Nonetheless, people do report adverse effects, ranging from headaches to chronic fatigue. In these cases, the problems generally go away when people stop using the sweeteners. So it's pretty easy to test whether or not artificial sweeteners are making you feel poorly. And if they are, the solution is simply to stop using them.

Do Artificial Sweeteners Help with Weight Loss?

The research on whether artificial sweeteners help you lose weight is mixed. Some studies have suggested that artificial sweeteners can increase your appetite, especially for sweets. Other studies have found that people who use artificial sweeteners lose more weight. As far as I can tell, the only time sugar substitutes seem to be helpful with weight management is when they are used in the context of a strict dietary regimen. Casual use of artificial sweeteners, on the other hand, is more often linked to weight gain. Unless you are paying close attention, you could end up unconsciously overcompensating for the calories you think you are saving by choosing artificially sweetened foods. My best advice is that all sweet-tasting foods, including artificially sweetened ones, should consumed in moderation.

The Different Types of Artificial Sweeteners

If the pros of artificial sweeteners outweigh the cons for you, here's a guide to the sugar substitutes found in most grocery stores.

ACESULFAME K—(Sunnett, Sweet One) Synthetic, zero-calorie sweetener, approximately two hundred times sweeter than sugar. It retains its sweetness when heated but has a bitter aftertaste. Commonly used in combination with other zero-calorie sweeteners to mask aftertaste.

ASPARTAME—(Equal, Nutrasweet) Zero-calorie sweetener synthesized from amino acids. About 200 times sweeter than sugar, but loses its sweetness when heated. Some bitter aftertaste.

ERYTHRITOL—(Swerve) Sugar alcohol produced from plant sugars. It's about 70 percent as sweet as sugar and contains a trivial amount of calories but does not affect blood sugar. Erythritol retains its sweetness when heated but tends to dehydrate baked goods. It has no aftertaste and a "cool" mouth feel.

What's a Sugar Alcohol?

Sugar alcohols aren't sugar (although they do taste sweet) and they aren't alcohol—at least, not the sort of alcohol that we imbibe in alcoholic beverages. Sugar alcohols include maltitol, xylitol, erythritol, sorbitol, and others—the "ol" ending usually signals a sugar alcohol. They are lower in calories than sugar but not calorie-free. In addition, because the shape of the molecule is slightly different than a true sugar, sugar alcohols do not cause an increase in blood sugar, which makes them helpful for diabetics. Overdoing it with sugar alcohols can cause temporary but unpleasant side effects such as diarrhea. A newer sugar alcohol called *erythritol* supposedly minimizes this effect.

SACCHARINE—(Sweet'N Low) Chemically synthesized zero-calorie sweetener about four hundred times sweetener than sugar. It retains its sweetness when heated but provides no browning. It has a bitter aftertaste.

STEVIA—A green herb whose leaves are extremely sweet but contain virtually no calories. Dried stevia leaves are about thirty times sweeter than sugar but have a strong herbal flavor. Stevia is usually refined and sold as an extremely concentrated powder or liquid, or cut with a filler like maltodextrin or inulin fiber to make it pour and measure more like regular sugar. It retains its sweetness when heated but has some aftertaste.

TRUVIA AND PUREVIA—Brand-name sweeteners containing a blend of stevia extracts and erythritol. Both are as sweet as sugar and retain their sweetness when heated, but they do not produce browning.

SUCRALOSE—(Splenda) Zero-calorie sweetener synthetized from sugar, about eight hundred times sweeter than sugar, with less aftertaste than saccharine, stevia, or aspartame. Retains sweetness when heated but does not brown.

Best Choice in Artificial Sweeteners

Most natural/safest: stevia, erythritol
Best (but not ideal) for baking: erythritol, sucralose
Least aftertaste: erythritol, sucralose

SALT

When shopping for salt at the grocery store, you'll have to choose between iodized and uniodized, sea salt, kosher salt, and gourmet salts. What are the differences?

The Different Types of Salt

TABLE SALT—May be harvested from rock salt, a natural salt deposit in the earth, or from evaporated seawater. Once it's been cleaned up and purified, there's no chemical or nutritional difference between the two.

SEA SALT—Always produced from seawater; crystals may be fine or coarse. The size of the salt crystal makes a difference in how you perceive the salt that you put *on* your food. Larger crystals sprinkled on a dish give a concentrated burst of saltiness and a little crunch that many people enjoy.

IODIZED SALT—Table or sea salt with added iodine, an essential nutrient. Iodized salt was proposed as an easy way to prevent iodine deficiency—and, for the most part, it has worked pretty well. Iodine deficiency is rare in industrialized countries. Some people don't like iodized salt because they feel that iodine adds a noticeable flavor. If you prefer not to use iodized salt, just be sure there are other sources of iodine in your diet. Vegetables can be a source of iodine, depending on the iodine content of the soil in which they're grown. Seafood and sea vegetables are other good sources. And many dairy farmers add iodine to the feed for the cows, so dairy products can be a good source of iodine. Even if you don't use iodized salt at home, a lot of processed and prepared foods are made with iodized salt. If these foods are in your diet, they are likely to be an additional source of iodine. Many multivitamins also include iodine.

KOSHER SALT—Has the same amount of sodium by weight as table and sea salt but only about half as much sodium per teaspoon. The big difference is the size and shape of the crystals, which are larger and flatter, as if you took a medium-coarse grain of salt and put it through a roller. The "fluffier" crystals take up more space so that less fits into the measuring spoon. As with sea salt, the size and shape of the crystal also makes a difference in how you perceive the saltiness. Because of the increased surface area of kosher salt crystals, they dissolve more readily on your tongue. For salt added during cooking, this wouldn't make any difference. But when sprinkling salt on top of a finished dish, you may find that using kosher salt gives you more flavor with less salt.

UNREFINED (GOURMET) SALT—Retains minerals and sediments that are usually filtered out of finished salt. Pink, gray, green, and lavender salts from exotic locales around the world are prized as gourmet ingredients but claims about the health benefits of unrefined salts should be taken with a grain of, well, salt. Unlike table salt, which contains only sodium, unrefined salts may also contain other minerals, such as potassium and magnesium, as well things like strontium, fluoride, and cadmium. There's also the chance that you're getting minerals you don't really want, like mercury or arsenic. Either way, however, we're talking about amounts that are measured in parts per million or fractions of a percent. Unrefined sea salts may be 5 to 10 percent lower in sodium than regular table salt.

LOW-SODIUM SALT ALTERNATIVES—These are mineral salts formed from potassium instead of sodium. Potassium chloride is a safe and natural option for those who need to avoid all sodium. It tastes salty, but can have a bitter or metallic aftertaste. You'll often find potassium chloride blended with various flavoring agents to create a better flavor profile.

Reducing Sodium: Reality Check

Keep in mind that 70 to 80 percent of sodium in most people's diets comes from packaged and prepared foods, including restaurant food. If you eat out a lot or you eat a lot of processed foods—things like canned soups, sauces, and vegetables, frozen dinners, deli meats, boxed meal kits, chips, snacks, and crackers—replacing the salt in your saltshaker with a low-sodium alternative is sort of like standing out in a driving rain storm and holding an umbrella over one knee.

If you're concerned about your sodium intake, start by cutting back on packaged and processed foods—which is where most of the sodium in your diet is coming from. If you do most of your own cooking using fresh whole foods, you're probably well within the general guidelines for sodium intake.

HERBS AND SPICES

Dried herbs and spices are another way to add flavor to your cooking without adding sodium. Along with an incredible variety of flavors, herbs and spices offer a vast array of nutritional and health benefits as well. Some of the most potent choices are highlighted in the box below, but my advice is to play the field.

Spices and dried herbs may seem as if they last forever but the volatile oils that give them their pungency are somewhat perishable. For maximum flavor and nutritional benefit, buy your herbs and spices in small quantities, store them away from heat and light in air-tight containers, and use them within a year.

Super Spices

Antioxidant activity: clove, allspice
Blood-sugar control: cinnamon
Anti-inflammatory activity: curry powder, turmeric, ginger, garlic
Appetite regulation: red pepper flakes, cayenne pepper

OILS

There are lots of different oils, produced from all kinds of fruits, vegetables, grains, nuts, and seeds. As you can see from the box, oils contain different proportions of mono- , poly- , and unsaturated fats. Although there's room for all three in a healthy diet, research suggests that you're better off when most of the fat in your diet is monounsaturated. Diets that are high in monounsaturated fats are linked to reduced risk of heart disease, cancer, and obesity.

Types of Fat in Oils

High in monounsaturated fat: hazelnut, olive, avocado, almond, canola

High in polyunsaturated fat: grapeseed, flaxseed, vegetable, walnut, soybean, vegetable, sesame

High in saturated fat: palm kernel, coconut

Of the oils that are high in monounsaturated fats, olive oil is also rich in polyphenols and antioxidants, which reduce inflammation and protect your cells against damage that can lead to cancer and heart disease. Cold-pressed, unfiltered, extra-virgin olive oil is highest in these compounds—which also contribute a lot of characteristic olivey flavor to the oil. Although I suggest that you use extra-virgin olive oil as your primary oil, there may be times when you want an oil with a little *less* flavor. You can buy "light olive oil" that's been filtered and refined to make it more neutral in flavor—at the expense of some of the polyphenols. For a completely neutral flavor, you can also choose canola oil, which obviously doesn't contain any of the special olive polyphenols but is equivalent in terms of monounsaturated fats. (See "The Canola Controversy" on page 72.)

The Canola Controversy

In some circles, canola oil has gotten a very bad reputation. It's said to be unnatural or even toxic. Canola oil is made from a type of rapeseed, which is a plant in the cabbage family, and is also related to turnips and mustard. That mustard relation may be the basis for the urban legend that rapeseed oil was used to make poisonous mustard gas in World War I. It wasn't.

In fact, rapeseed oil was used for centuries as a cooking oil in Asia. In modern times, it fell out of favor as a food oil, especially in the West. First, it has a bitter taste that most people find unpalatable. And second, it's naturally high in a fatty acid called erucic acid; some early animal studies raised concerns about the effects of consuming large amounts of this fatty acid.

Subsequent research has now largely put to rest most of the health concerns about erucic acid—or at least put them into perspective. But long before that happened, some Canadian growers solved the problem a different way. They simply bred a type of rapeseed that was low in erucic acid. In the process, they also reduced the bitter taste that made rapeseed oil unpalatable. The seed they bred produced a light, flavorless oil that was very high in the healthiest types of fats: the monounsaturated fats and omega-3 fatty acids. The Canadian growers appeared to have a highly marketable product on their hands—in all ways but one. "Low-erucic rapeseed oil" just didn't have that winning ring to it. So they coined—and trademarked—the term *canola oil* to identify this new cultivar, or breed, of rapeseed oil.

Just how did these growers manage to produce rapeseed oil that was low in erucic acid? Well, I guess you could say that canola oil was genetically modified. But we're not talking about inserting genes from a fruit fly into a rapeseed plant. The agricultural engineers who produced canola oil went about it the good, old-fashioned way that we've been genetically modifying plants for hundreds of years. They selectively bred the plants to enhance certain desirable characteristics and suppress others. I've heard people say that they won't consume canola oil because it didn't exist fifty years ago. That's true.

Neither did Fuji apples or seedless watermelons. They were both produced using the same methods that produced canola oil. If you feel comfortable eating these foods, then canola oil shouldn't present any special issues.

Long after canola oil was developed with selective breeding, a much different kind of genetic modification arrived on the scene. Bioengineering allows scientists to take individual genes from plants, viruses, bacteria, or other organisms, and splice them into another organism's genetic code—and this is what most people are worried about when they talk about genetically modified organisms, or GMOs, entering the food supply.

Perhaps the most notorious example of genetically engineered foods are strains of corn, soy, and, yes, canola that have been modified to withstand certain herbicides and other agricultural chemicals. The agribusiness giant Monsanto, for example, has produced seeds that have been genetically modified to allow them to survive applications of Monsanto's weedkiller, Roundup. These Roundup Ready seeds allow farmers to apply Roundup to their fields without killing the crops. Farmers are now freed from more labor-intensive forms of weed control and yields have exploded. It's working out well for Monsanto, too. First, it allows them to do something rather extraordinary—get a patent on a seed. Second, farmers who buy Roundup Ready seeds also have to buy Roundup brand weedkiller, because the seeds have been engineered to withstand only Monsanto's herbicides—another brand of weedkiller might kill them.

Like it or not, genetically engineered foods have become extremely common, which is a source of great controversy and concern. Some people worry that tampering with nature will produce unforeseen consequences. They may be right. So, I can certainly understand if you want to avoid plants that have been produced using genetic engineering. You can still find canola (and soy and corn) products that specify that they are GMO free—and buying these products is one small way to help ensure that genetically engineered crops aren't the only plants we have left fifty years from now.

Omega-3 and Omega-6 Fats

Polyunsaturated fats can be divided into two families: omega-3 and omega-6. Fish, walnuts, flax, chia, and hemp seeds are all good sources of omega-3 fats. Vegetable oils like corn, soybean, and peanut oils are high in omega-6. Omega-6 fats aren't bad for you; they are just as essential as omega-3s. But your body works best when you have a balanced intake of omega-3s and omega-6s, and most of us get a lot more omega-6 than omega-3. One way to improve the balance is to avoid oils that are high in omega-6, including corn, soybean, peanut, sunflower, and safflower oils.

How Many Oils Do You Need?

One or two all-purpose oils like olive and canola will cover the majority of your cooking needs. You'll also find a variety of "specialty" oils that are used in small quantities as flavoring accents. For example, you might use a teaspoon of toasted sesame oil in an Asian dish or some walnut or hazelnut oil in a salad dressing. If you do a lot of cooking, you may accumulate quite a collection of these special oils, but try to avoid buying more than you'll be able to use up with in a couple of months. Nut and seed oils go rancid fairly quickly—and rancid oils are not safe to consume. Keeping them in the refrigerator will preserve them a while longer. Always give oil a sniff before using it to check for the characteristic stale or sour odor that signals rancidity. If there's any doubt about whether an oil has gone rancid, it's best to discard it.

What Oil Labels Mean

Here are some terms that describe how the oil was produced and the advantages of each. When you don't see any of these terms on the label, you can assume the oil was chemically extracted and refined at high temperatures.

COLD-PRESSED—Oil is mechanically extracted at low temperatures to minimize degradation of delicate flavors and/or nutrients. Cold-pressed oils are generally unrefined (virgin).

EXPELLER PRESSED—Oil is extracted under high pressure but without the use of chemicals. Expeller pressed may be refined or unrefined (virgin).

ORGANIC—Oils are produced from plants grown without synthetic pesticides and herbicides. Not only will the oil itself be free of residues from these chemicals, but choosing organic products reduces the use of agricultural pesticides, which benefits the larger environment. Organic oils may be refined or unrefined (virgin).

REFINED—Oil is filtered to remove impurities, including nutrients and other compounds, which increases the smoke point of the oil. Refined oils are less flavorful and not as nutritious but better for high-heat cooking.

TOASTED—Oils are made by toasting nuts or seeds before the oil is pressed, intensifying the flavor. Toasted oils are generally unrefined (virgin) and may be filtered or unfiltered.

UNFILTERED—Oil contains minute particles from the fruit or nut it was pressed from, preserving flavor and nutrients.

VIRGIN—Unrefined oil. It may be filtered or unfiltered.

Which Oils Are Best for High-heat Cooking?

Both olive and canola oil are fine to use for brief or moderate-heat cooking like sauteing, roasting, or baking. If you're going to be cooking at higher temperatures, such as frying, you'll want an oil with a higher smoke point. Palm kernel and coconut oils are very stable at high heat. You can also buy canola oil that is specially refined for high-heat applications. I suggest you avoid frying with vegetable oils that are high in polyunsaturated fats—even those with high smoke points. Heating polyunsaturated oils can cause harmful compounds to form.

Best Choices in Oil

Best choice for overall nutrition: extra-virgin olive oil
Best choice for neutral flavor: canola (expeller pressed)
Best choice for gourmet touches: hazelnut, walnut
Best choice for high-heat cooking: palm kernel, high-heat canola

---

Shortening

Vegetable shortening, such as Crisco, was originally made from of partially hydrogenated vegetable oil and was extremely high in trans fats. Once the dangers of trans fat became widely known, the product was reformulated and because it now contains less than half a gram of trans fats per serving (1 tablespoon), Crisco can legally claim 0 grams of trans fat per serving. If you read the ingredient list, however, you'll see that it still contains partially hydrogenated vegetable oil, which means that it still contains trans fats.

Although olive or canola oil would be a better choice nutritionally, substituting oil for shortening may change the texture of some recipes. (As bad as it is for you, shortening produces flaky, tender baked goods and crisp fried foods.) Spectrum Naturals carries an organic shortening made with 100 percent palm kernel oil. Although it's high in saturated fat, palm kernel oil shortening or butter would be preferable to shortening containing partially hydrogenated oil.

THE QUICK AND DIRTY SECRET

Choose shortening made without partially hydrogenated vegetable oil—or substitute butter.

Mayonnaise

Classic mayonnaise is made by incorporating oil into egg yolks, and labeling regulations dictate that in order for a commercial product to be called "mayonnaise," it must contain eggs. Products without eggs are labeled "imitation mayonnaise." Given that the cholesterol in eggs is not the threat we once thought it was, you can choose whichever you like better. Either way, check the ingredient list to see what type of oil is used. Many commercial products use soybean oil, which is high in omega-6 fats. Mayonnaise made with canola or olive oil, both of which are high in monounsaturated fat, is a better choice. Because it is mostly fat, regular mayonnaise (both real and imitation) is relatively high in calories—about 100 calories per table-spoon. Fat-free versions, on the other hand, replace the fat with sugar, gums, gels, and other additives. Reduced fat or light mayonnaise offers a reasonable compromise for those concerned about calories; they're about half the calories and don't contain as many artificial ingredients.

THE QUICK AND DIRTY SECRET

Mayonnaise made with canola or olive oil is a better choice than mayonnaise made with soybean oil. If calories are a concern, choose light (not fat-free) mayo and look for the brand with the fewest artificial ingredients.

VINEGARS

Vinegar can be made from just about anything: wine, fruit juice, grains—even wood! It's made through a two-step fermentation process in which sugars are converted to alcohol and then the alcohol is further converted to acetic acid—which is the compound that gives vinegar that unmistakable sour or tart taste. Vinegar is generally very low in calories, and with the wide array of distinctive varieties and flavors available it's a great way to add flavor to marinades, salad dressings, and sauces. When used in marinades, vinegar also helps tenderize meats.

Different Types of Vinegar

Here's a guide to the most common types of vinegar.

DISTILLED—Sharp and pungent, distilled vinegar is not very palatable. It's most useful in pickling and also makes a great household cleaner and fruit and vegetable wash.

CIDER—Made from fermented apples, cider vinegar has a high acidity and a fruity flavor. Too aggressive for most vinaigrettes, it's good in marinades, condiments (like chutney), and to cut the heaviness of mayonnaise-based dressings (like coleslaw).

WINE—Made from both red and white wine, wine vinegar is a little milder than cider or distilled vinegar. It works well in vinaigrettes. As with actual wine, it's often worth it to spend a little more on wine-based vinegars.

MALT—Made from malted barley, malt vinegar, has a distinctive yeasty flavor. It's similar in potency to cider vinegar and can be used interchangeably.

BALSAMIC—Sweet and fruity, balsamic vinegar is higher in sugar and calories than most vinegars. However, its low acidity means that salad dressings made with it require a lot less oil. Balsamic vinegar can be reduced (concentrated) and used as a glaze for meat, drizzled over roasted vegetables, or even poured on top of sliced fruit.

RICE OR RICE WINE—Mild and slightly sweet, rice vinegar has a smooth, mellow flavor. Its low acidity means that salad dressings made with it usually require less oil.

SEASONED RICE VINEGAR—This is rice vinegar with a small amount of sugar and salt added to it. It can be used right out of the bottle to dress cucumber salad, mixed with soy sauce for a quick Asian dipping sauce, or used in vinaigrettes.

HERBAL—Distilled, wine, or cider vinegar, infused with garlic, tarragon, rosemary, or other herbs. Use in marinades or salad dressings for added interest.

FRUIT—Berry, currant, or other fruit vinegars are sweeter and less acidic (similar to balsamic) and lend distinctive flavors to salad dressings and sauces.

THE QUICK AND DIRTY SECRET

Vinegar is a healthy way to add flavor to foods. If you're trying to keep it simple, cider and balsamic vinegar will cover most of your needs.

LET'S TAKE A CLOSER LOOK

Does Vinegar Burn Fat?

Vinegar has been touted as a weight-loss aid for ages and there is actually some science to back up the lore. Acetic acid is the substance that gives vinegar its characteristic tart or sour quality. This compound also seems to activate certain genes that cause one's body to store less fat around the waist and deposit it more evenly around the body. As if that weren't enough, acetic acid also appears to increase thermogenesis, causing the body's engine to run a little hotter—burning more calories in the process. As good as all this sounds, these effects are unlikely to translate into substantial weight loss—especially given the fact that vinegar is consumed in relatively small quantities. But there is one more way that vinegar might help you battle the bulge. Research shows that adding vinegar to a meal slows down the speed at which the carbohydrates are converted to sugar in your bloodstream. That can help ratchet down your appetite and even reduce your risk of developing diabetes.

Bottled Salad Dressing

Bottled salad dressings are convenient but they're often unnecessarily high in sugar and salt. In general, the thinner, oil-and-vinegar-based (vinaigrette) dressings are healthier than the thick, gloppy ones. And because the excess tends to run off the salad, they usually add a lot fewer calories, even when they're not "low-calorie." Look for brands with short lists of recognizable ingredients—such as oil and vinegar rather than maltodextrin and xanthan gum. If you enjoy the taste of blue cheese, skip the Roquefort dressing and crumble a little blue cheese on top of your salad instead.

THE QUICK AND DIRTY SECRET

Choose vinaigrette-style dressings made with recognizable ingredients. Avoid thick, creamy salad dressings and those with lots of artificial additives.

NUTS AND SEEDS

Nuts and seeds have a lot going for them nutritionally. They are rich in antioxidants, fiber, and heart-healthy fats. They also contain nutrients called plant sterols, which help to lower LDL (or "bad") cholesterol. They're portable and relatively nonperishable, which makes them handy for healthy snacks. They can also be an important source of protein for vegetarians. As you can see in the box below, almost every common nut and seed has a particular nutritional strength, so it makes sense to enjoy the variety. When shopping for nuts and seeds, avoid the "honey-roasted" or "smokehouse" varieties, which are extravagantly high in sodium, artificial flavorings, and other additives. Dry-roasted, lightly salted nuts and seeds are a better option. Raw, unsalted nuts and seeds are your best choice. To enhance the flavor of raw nuts and seeds, toast them briefly in a dry skillet, shaking often to prevent scorching.

Best Choices in Nuts and Seeds

Higher in protein: peanuts, pumpkin seeds
Higher in fiber: chia, flax, almonds
Higher in phytosterols (cholesterol-lowering compounds): sesame, sunflower, pistachio
Higher in omega-3s: flax, chia, walnuts
Higher in calcium: sesame, chia, almonds
Lower in fat and calories: chestnuts, pumpkin, cashews

Nut and Seed Butters

Nut and seed butters, such as peanut butter, almond butter, cashew butter, and sunflower seed butter, are another great way to enjoy these nutritious foods, but look for brands with a short list of ingredients. Ideally, they will contain little more than the nut or seed and maybe a bit of salt. Avoid brands that include sugar, hydrogenated oils, and other additives. Separated oil is the sign of a minimally processed nut butter. Though it may be a bit of a hassle to have to stir it back in, it indicates that the fats have not been chemically altered.

All nut and seed butters are naturally high in fat. Although reduced-fat versions may seem like a good idea, what they add is often less desirable than what they subtract. Reduced-fat nut butters usually have more sugar, salt, and other processed ingredients like defatted peanut flour. Often, they're not even that much lower in calories than regular versions. If anything, replacing calories from healthy fats with calories from sugar is a step in the wrong direction.

ALLERGIC TO PEANUTS? TRY SOY-NUT BUTTER!—If a peanut allergy prevents you from enjoying peanut butter, soy-nut butter may be a good substitute. Despite their name, peanuts aren't actually nuts at all—they're legumes, as are soybeans. Soy-nut butter has a nutritional profile, texture, and flavor that's similar to peanut butter. Although the two are in the same botanical family, most people with peanut allergies are not allergic to soy. Though soy is a healthy choice, it's a good idea to limit your intake of soy foods to three servings a day. (For more on soy, see Is Soy Dangerous on page 22.)

THE QUICK AND DIRTY SECRET

Look for butters made with ground nuts or seeds and not much else.

DRIED FRUIT

Although not quite as nutritious as fresh fruit, dried fruit has a long shelf life and makes a convenient, portable snack. It makes a good alternative to processed sweets and a healthy addition to baked treats such as Best Fruit and Nut Bars (recipe on page 206). Dried fruits are usually made with sulfites, which are antioxidants (preservatives) that keep the fruit from turning brown. Sulfites can cause reactions in some people—causing symptoms similar to an asthma attack or allergic reaction. People with sulfite sensitivity should avoid dried fruits or look for "unsulfured" fruit. However, if you are not sensitive to sulfites, they are not harmful and there's no reason to avoid them. Look for dried fruit without added sugars or oils.

Best Choices in Dried Fruit

High in antioxidants: blueberries, cherries, apricots
Higher in fiber: persimmons, apples, figs
Lower in sugar: apricots, prunes, figs
Higher in iron: apricots, prunes

DRIED BEANS

Dried beans are another good staple to keep on hand because of their nutritional value and great versatility. High in both protein and fiber, they can be combined with vegetables, pasta, grains, and seasonings for an infinite variety of nutritious soups, casseroles, salads, and meatless main courses.

You'll find dried beans in every size and color, each with its own distinct attributes. Small black or red beans keep their shape and are great in soups or with rice. Speckled pinto beans have a creamy texture that makes them great for bean dips or burrito filling. Large white cannellini beans have a meaty heartiness that stands up well to pasta. Like beans, split peas and lentils are high in fiber and protein and come in a similar array of colors and varieties. One advantage to peas and lentils is that they cook much more quickly, which is great for last-minute meals. The following box shows some of the nutritional highlights of various types of beans but the differences are relatively minor.

Best Choices in Beans and Legumes

Higher in protein: white (by a small amount)
Higher in fiber: navy, pinto, black, cranberry
Lower in calories and carbohydrates: fava, lentil, split pea
Higher in iron: white, lentil, garbanzo,
Higher in folic acid: cranberry, lentil, garbanzo, pinto

CANNED VEGGIES

As a general rule, frozen vegetables are more nutritious than canned vegetables—and they usually have no added salt, which allows you to control how much sodium is in your dishes and your diet. The texture and flavor of frozen vegetables and dried beans is usually superior to their canned counterparts as well.

However, it can be handy to have a few canned vegetables on hand. Canned beans are helpful for those times that you don't have time to cook from scratch. I also always keep canned tomatoes in the cupboard. Other things that come in handy for recipes are olives, corn, water chestnuts, and artichoke hearts.

Are Canned Goods Safe?

Recently, there have been concerns about the chemical bisphenol A, or BPA, which is used as a lining in virtually all canned foods. BPA forms a barrier between the food and the metal of the can, which helps keep the can from corroding. The problem is that it leaches into the foods and gets into our bodies, where some fear it might have harmful effects on hormones or reproductive health. The primary concern is infants, small children, and pregnant and nursing mothers. Steps have already been taken to remove BPA from baby bottles.

As of this writing, BPA is still being used in canned goods while the FDA conducts further research to verify its safety. In the meantime, many consumers have decided they'd rather err on the side of caution. A few companies offer BPA-free canned goods. Vegetables preserved in glass jars or cardboard boxes (also called aseptic packaging) are other options. The highest levels of BPA are found in canned tomato products, due to the high acid level of tomatoes.

To reduce BPA exposure, use fresh or frozen vegetables and dried beans rather than canned vegetables and beans whenever possible. Buy tomatoes in glass jars or aseptic packaging.

WHAT'S THE GAME PLAN?

Your Shopping Game Plan for Pantry Staples

Meals that you prepare at home will almost always be nutritionally superior to anything you could carry out or have delivered. Keeping your pantry stocked with the basics will ensure that you always have what you need to put together healthy meals. For the most part, pantry staples are nonperishable, so you can buy enough to last a couple of months and restock as needed. Whenever you start to run low on dried beans, pasta, olive oil, or canned tomatoes, make a note so that you can stock up on your next grocery trip.

Even nonperishable foods lose nutrients and quality with extended storage, so you don't want things sitting around in your cupboard for years. Some rainy Saturday, go through your cupboards and throw away any food that is past its expiration date or that has been in there so long you can't remember when you bought it. The list below shows how long different nonperishables keep. Use it as a guide for how much to buy.

Use within three to six months: oil, flour, nuts, seeds, cereal
Use within a year: canned goods, whole intact grains, dried fruits, pasta, spices, sweeteners, dried beans

Everything Else Is Optional

Having gathered your fresh foods and restocked your pantry, you could theoretically leave the store and have everything you need! But there are whole aisles we haven't gone near, including a staggering array of snacks, treats, beverages, prepared foods, convenience foods, and ready-to-eat meals. In the next chapter, we'll talk about all of these optional items.

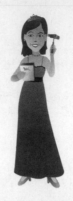

CHAPTER THREE

Packaged and Prepared Foods

AT THE GROCERY store, processed, packaged, and prepared foods occupy most of the shelf space and fresh, whole foods are in the minority. Ideally, your grocery cart—and day—will be exactly the opposite, with more fresh, whole foods and fewer processed, packaged, and prepared foods. Compared with meals you make yourself, processed foods tend to contain less of the good stuff (like nutrients) and more of the bad stuff (like excess sodium, sugar, calories, and additives).

However, there is no denying the convenience of ready-made meals, especially when schedules are tight. You'll find ready-to-eat options throughout the grocery store, from canned soups to frozen dinners to dehydrated mixes. And fortunately, there are some newer brands that cater to health-conscious consumers, so it's become a bit easier to find healthier options. In this chapter, I won't be making the sort of "Best Choices" recommendations that I did in the last two chapters. The number of options is simply too vast and changing too fast for that to be practical. Instead, I'll give you some tips on how to make wise choices when selecting packaged foods. Regardless of the brand or format, however, the secret to finding the best choices is in learning how to decode the information on the package.

PACKAGED FOODS

Keep in mind that the information on the *front* of the package is advertising. The manufacturer can't say anything that's untrue, of course. But they're certainly going to put the best possible spin on things. They're going to draw attention to the fact that the product is Organic! High in fiber! Gluten-free! You're not going to see little starbursts proclaiming Lots of preservatives! High in sodium! Fortified with synthetic vitamins to replace what got lost in processing! To get the whole story, you need to turn the package over and look for the ingredient list and Nutrition Facts label.

Ingredients Should Be Foods, Not Chemicals

Start by scanning the ingredient list. Do you see ingredients you recognize as foods? Or does it read like the inventory of a chemistry lab? Compare, for example, the ingredient lists of these two brands of frozen veggie burgers. Which one looks more like a recipe to you?

BOCA BURGER'S ALL-AMERICAN MEATLESS SOY BURGERS	DR. PRAEGER'S CALIFORNIA STYLE VEGGIE BURGERS
Water, Soy Protein Concentrate, Mild Reduced Fat Cheddar, Wheat Gluten, Salt, Soy Sauce, Cheese Flavor, Dried Onion, Yeast Extract, Autolyzed Yeast Extract, Partially Hydrogenated Cottonseed and Soybean Oil, Defatted Wheat Germ, Sesame Oil, Caramel Color, Methylcellulose, Dextrose, Lactic Acid, Partially Hydrogenated Soybean Oil	Carrots, Onions, String beans, Soybeans, Zucchini, Oat Bran, Peas, Spinach, Expeller Pressed Canola Oil, Broccoli, Textured Soy Flour, Corn, Oat Fiber, Red Pepper, Arrowroot, Corn Meal, Corn Starch, Garlic, Salt, Parsley, Black Pepper, All Natural Vegetable Gum

Almost all of the ingredients on the right are foods that I regularly cook with myself. By comparison, the ingredient list on the left looks more like instructions for a chemistry experiment. I can only find six ingredients that I've ever used in a recipe—including water and salt.

I'm not against chemistry, by the way. It's not that autolyzed yeast extract or methylcellulose are harmful. Both, in fact, are perfectly harmless. (I can't say the same for partially hydrogenated soybean oil.) But in what aisle of the grocery store would you look for them? Where would you find the dextrose or lactic acid or caramel color? A long list of ingredients that you'd have difficulty finding in a grocery store is the hallmark of a highly processed, industrially produced food. No matter how many vitamins they spray on at the end of the conveyor belt, these manufactured products can never match the nutritional value of real food.

In the previous two chapters, I highlighted the healthiest fresh foods and ingredients in the grocery store. These are the foods you want to see in ingredient lists on packaged foods. When you see olive oil instead of soybean oil or honey instead of high-fructose corn syrup, or herbs instead of artificial flavors, it suggests that the manufacturers are using the same type of ingredients that you'd choose if you were doing the cooking.

Remember as well that ingredients are listed in order by the amount used, from the biggest percentage to the smallest. I'm impressed, for example, that eight out of the first ten ingredients in the Dr. Praeger's burgers are vegetables. By contrast, I have to get a third of the way down the ingredient list for the Boca Burgers before hitting the first (and only) thing that looks sort of like a vegetable. It's a good sign when the ingredient list contains things you recognize—things you'd be able to find elsewhere in the grocery store. It's even better when the ingredients that reflect the kinds of foods you want to emphasize in your diet.

Trans Fats: The Good, the Bad, and the Invisible

Most people have heard that trans fats are bad news—in particular, the partially hydrogenated vegetable oils used in packaged and processed foods. These are fats that have been chemically rearranged to increase their shelf life. Although this process makes them more useful to manufacturers, it also makes them more destructive to the human body. The trans fats in partially hydrogenated oils clog arteries and provoke inflammation and cell damage. There are even studies suggesting that they are more fattening than other fats, even though they contain the same number of calories.

But not all trans fats are human-made. Small amounts of trans fats occur naturally in dairy and beef. These natural trans fats don't seem to have the same damaging health effects as the human-made trans fats that you find in hydrogenated vegetable oils. In fact, preliminary research suggests that some of the naturally occurring trans fats in dairy may actually be beneficial!

For several years now, trans fats have been listed on the Nutrition Facts label of packaged foods. Unfortunately, there's no way to distinguish between harmful, human-made trans fats and harmless, natural trans fats. What's worse, labeling laws allow manufacturers to "round down," meaning that foods containing a half gram of trans fats per serving or less may be labeled "0 grams trans fat" or trans-fat free. If you're trying to avoid human-made trans fats (which I think is a very good idea), your best bet is to check the ingredient list and avoid foods that list "partially hydrogenated" oils.

What about Fully Hydrogenated Oil?

If an oil is fully hydrogenated, it no longer contains any trans fats. Instead, it has been chemically transformed into saturated fat. Because it contains no trans fats, fully hydrogenated oil is not as harmful as partially hydrogenated oil—but not as healthy as mono-unsaturated fats, either.

THE QUICK AND DIRTY SECRET

Avoid packaged foods that contain partially hydrogenated oils.

The Many Aliases of Sugar

One big reason that sugar intake is so out of control these days is that sugar is added—in one form or another—to virtually every packaged and processed food. The more processed foods you include in your diet, the faster these hidden sugars can add up. When scanning ingredient lists, watch for words that signal added sugar:

> Sugar (beet, brown, cane, confectioner's, date, demerara, grape, invert, malt, powdered, raw, turbinado)
> Cane (crystals, juice, syrup)
> Syrup (malt, corn, maple, cane, high fructose, glucose/ fructose, refiner's, rice, sorghum)
> Words ending in "ose" (glucose, fructose, sucrose, dextrose, maltose)
> Maltodextrin
> Honey
> Molasses
> Malt (syrup, barley, sugar)
> Concentrated fruit juice (pear, grape)

Be particularly alert for ingredient lists that contain sugar in several different forms. Using small amounts of several types of sweeteners allows the manufacturers to bury these ingredients farther down the list—even though sugar may still be one of the principal ingredients.

LET'S TAKE A CLOSER LOOK

Is High Fructose Corn Syrup Worse than Sugar?

You may have heard that the United States—and most of the Western world—has a growing obesity problem. One likely reason is that we're consuming far more sugar than we used to. When consumed in these prodigious quantities, refined sugar seems to affect appetite and metabolism in ways that promote obesity. Lately, there's been a lot of focus on high-fructose corn syrup, a refined sweetener that's widely used in processed foods and beverages. But the problem isn't that it's that much worse for you than other forms of sugar—or even that it's particularly high in fructose (it contains roughly the same amount of fructose as cane sugar). If high-fructose corn syrup is to blame for rising obesity rates, it is simply because it has become the primary source of sugar in the modern diet.

Avoiding high-fructose corn syrup can be an effective way to reduce your sugar intake. What's more, foods made with high-fructose corn syrup tend to be highly processed and without a lot of nutritional value. You're better off without them! But if you simply replace these foods with things made with cane sugar or other sweeteners instead, you won't have accomplished much.

The goal is to reduce your consumption of all sweeteners, even the natural ones.

HOW TO USE THE NUTRITION FACTS LABEL

After you've vetted the ingredient list, you also want to check the Nutrition Facts label to see how the food adds (or subtracts) from your nutrition goals from the day.

Serving Size

First, check how many servings the package contains. You'd be amazed at how many things that appear to be packaged as single servings are listed as two or three servings on the Nutrition Facts label. If you overlook this critical fact, you could easily be consuming far more calories than you mean to.

Calories

To get a quick estimate of what percentage of the day's calorie intake a food represents, knock off the last digit and then divide in half. For example, if a serving contains 180 calories, it represents about 9 percent of your daily allowance $(18 \div 2 = 9)$. That's sounds right for a snack but might be a little skimpy for an entire meal. On the other hand, a 560 calorie item—more than a quarter of the day's allowance—is probably a little much for an appetizer.

Daily Values

The Nutrition Facts label will also tell you how much fat, cholesterol, sodium, carbohydrate, fiber, and protein a food contains. To shed some light on what these numbers signify, the label also tells you what percentage of the Daily Value these amounts represent. The Daily Values are based on the average needs of a healthy adult with a 2,000 calorie diet. Even if this one-size-fits-all guideline isn't a perfect fit for *you*, these numbers are still useful.

Balancing the Numbers

The Daily Values (DVs) are not meant to be the last word in how much or little of each nutrient you should be taking in. Instead, use them as a quick way to gauge whether a ready-to-eat option makes a balanced meal. Here are some of the things I look for:

PROTEIN (% DV) EQUAL TO OR GREATER THAN CARBOHYDRATE (% DV)—As I'll talk more about in part 2, there's a fairly broad range of what's acceptable in terms of protein and carbohydrate intake. I think of the DV for protein (50 grams) as a recommended *minimum* and the DV for carbohydrates (300 grams) as a recommended *maximum*. Accordingly, I like to see meals where the % DV for protein is equal to or greater than the % DV for carbohydrate.

Quick Tip: The Daily Value for protein is not always included on the Nutrition Facts label. To calculate the percent Daily Value for protein, double the amount of protein grams. For example: If a serving contains 10 grams of protein, it provides 20 percent of the Daily Value for protein.

FIBER (% DV) EQUAL OR GREATER TO CARBOHYDRATE (% DV)— Fiber slows down the digestion of carbohydrates, which is generally a good thing. Slower digestion and absorption means that your blood-sugar levels stay steadier and you don't get hungry again as quickly. If a food is high in carbohydrates, it should also be high in fiber. A good rule of thumb is to look for foods where the % DV of fiber is equal to or greater than the % DV of carbohydrates.

SUGAR (g) NOT MORE THAN FIBER (g)—The carbohydrates in a food can be broken down into fiber, sugar, and starch. In addition to telling you how many grams of total carbohydrates a serving provides, the label also tells you how much of that total is fiber and sugar (everything else is starch). Most people tend to have too much sugar and not enough fiber in their diets. Avoiding foods that have more sugar than fiber will help you stay on target.

Stay Within Your Budget

The Daily Values can also help you budget your intake of things like sodium. For example, rather than choose a food that packs 60 percent of the Daily Value for sodium into a single serving, it might be wise to budget your sodium allowance more evenly throughout the day.

The Nutrition Facts Label: Putting It All Together

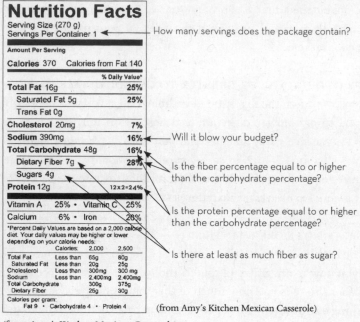

Nutrition Facts

Serving Size (270 g)
Servings Per Container 1 ◄——— How many servings does the package contain?

Amount Per Serving

Calories 370   Calories from Fat 140

	% Daily Value*
Total Fat 16g	**25%**
Saturated Fat 5g	**25%**
Trans Fat 0g	
Cholesterol 20mg	**7%**
Sodium 390mg	**16%** ◄——— Will it blow your budget?
Total Carbohydrate 48g	**16%**
Dietary Fiber 7g	**28%**
Sugars 4g	
Protein 12g	12x2=24%

Is the fiber percentage equal to or higher than the carbohydrate percentage?

Is the protein percentage equal to or higher than the carbohydrate percentage?

Is there at least as much fiber as sugar?

Vitamin A	25%	• Vitamin C	25%
Calcium	6%	• Iron	26%

*Percent Daily Values are based on a 2,000 calorie diet. Your daily values may be higher or lower depending on your calorie needs.

	Calories:	2,000	2,500
Total Fat	Less than	65g	80g
Saturated Fat	Less than	20g	25g
Cholesterol	Less than	300mg	300 mg
Sodium	Less than	2,400mg	2,400mg
Total Carbohydrate		300g	375g
Dietary Fiber		25g	30g

Calories per gram:
Fat 9 • Carbohydrate 4 • Protein 4

(from Amy's Kitchen Mexican Casserole)

(from Amy's Kitchen Mexican Casserole)

MEALS TO GO

These days, most grocery stores also double as takeout counters, with a wide array of prepared dishes. For people on the go, prepared foods from the deli counter can be awfully convenient. However, the convenience comes at a cost. Like restaurant food, prepared foods from the grocery tend to be higher in salt, fat, and sugar than foods you'd make for yourself. And because there is usually no Nutrition Facts label for these foods, there is nothing to provide a reality check on things like calories or serving size.

Unlike at a restaurant, however, you have the advantage of being able to see the food at the prepared food counter before you order. Use that to your advantage. Dishes that look slick with oil, are smothered in creamy sauce, swimming in gravy, or encrusted with crispy coatings and toppings are usually not the best picks. Instead, look for the simpler preparations. Grilled meats, fruit- and vegetable-heavy sides, and broth-based soups are good choices. And don't be afraid to ask questions. Many grocery stores have nutrition and ingredient information for their deli items available on request. Some also offer salads made with low-fat mayonnaise or sour cream. If you don't see them, let the store know you'd be interested in lighter options.

SWEET AND SALTY TREATS

I'm sure this won't come as a big surprise, but chips, pretzels, cookies, crackers, and desserts don't add much to the nutritional quality of your diet. They're mostly a source of excess calories, sodium, and sugar. If you're doing every else right—eating your vegetables, getting enough fiber and protein, choosing healthy fats and whole grains, and so on—the occasional treat isn't going to torpedo your efforts. The problem for most people (including me) is that these foods can be very seductive. "Bet you can't eat just one!" is more than an ad slogan; it pretty much sums up the problem with sweet and salty treats. You often end up eating more than you mean to.

Unless you have an iron will, I suggest that you don't test your willpower by keeping a lot of munchies and sweets around the house. This is one case where the large value pack is not the best choice. If snack foods are occupying a large percentage of your grocery cart, it's a good sign that they're too big a part of your diet. You should buy these foods exactly the way you should eat them—occasionally and in small quantities.

As a general rule, extras shouldn't make up more than about 10 to 15 percent of your total calories. In practical terms, that means maybe one extra for every five servings of vegetables—not the other way around.

Beware of the Health Halo

Deep down, you know that corn chips and cookies aren't healthy choices. But what about the corn chips with flaxseeds and gluten-free cookies over in the healthy foods aisle? People often overestimate the nutritional value of a food that's labeled "whole-grain" or "gluten-free." Or, they underestimate the negative impact of a food because it contains a healthful ingredient like flaxseed. This is known as the "health halo effect."

My favorite illustration of this effect is an experiment John Tierney did a couple of years ago in Brooklyn. He stopped a bunch of people on the street, showed them a photograph of a meal from a chain restaurant—one of those crunchy Asian chicken salads and a soda—and asked them to estimate how many calories the meal contained. On average, people estimated that the meal contained about 1,000 calories, which was a little high. It actually contained a little over 900 calories.

Then he stopped some more people and showed them a photo of the same salad and soda, *plus* two crackers that were labeled "trans-fat free." Despite the fact that the crackers actually added a hundred calories to the meal, the average calorie estimate for the meal with the crackers was about 800 calories—*two hundred calories less than the average estimate for same meal without the crackers*. The health halo conferred by two little words—trans-fat free—not only canceled out the calories in the crackers themselves, it erased a hundred calories from the salad sitting next to them—at least in people's minds.

Don't fall prey to the same magical thinking. By all means, read labels and look for things made with real foods instead of highly processed ingredients. Compare nutrition facts labels to find options that are lower in sodium and sugar and higher in fiber. Just remember that chips, crackers, cookies, ice cream, and other snacks and treats are still extras—even if they are made with green tea or goji berries or air-dried sea salt.

Is Microwave Popcorn a Healthy Snack?

As snack foods go, popcorn has a lot going for it. It's a whole-grain food, it's high in fiber, low in fat and sugar. In fact, I consider it to be one of the healthiest snack options around. But I am not a big fan of microwave popcorn products. Chemicals from the bags can turn into dangerous fumes when they're heated. Microwave popcorn is often sky-high in sodium and the artificial flavorings and colorings are a real turnoff, too. Plus, the cheapskate in me can't get over the

KITCHEN TIP

Microwave Popcorn for Cheapskates

Add three tablespoons of kernels to a brown paper lunch bag. Fold down the top half-inch of the bag two or three times. Place the bag on its side in microwave and hit the "popcorn" setting. Stay close to the microwave and stop it as soon as popping slows. (Popcorn burns quickly.) Immediately dump the popped corn into a large bowl. Pop another three tablespoons of corn, using the same bag. Meanwhile, heat one tablespoon of butter over low heat in a small saucepan or measuring cup. When melted, add one tablespoon extra-virgin olive oil to the butter, swirl briefly to mix, and drizzle the mixture over the popped corn. Toss to mix and salt to taste. Makes one large bowl.

Quick Tip: I've found that the "bow-tie-guy" brand and the organic popcorn from my health food store seem to pop up better than the cheaper generic brands. Even when you spring for the premium kernels, it's still a bargain compared with packaged microwave popcorn!

fact that for what you spend for three little oversalted bags, you can buy enough popcorn to fill a small room. See my recipe for cheap, chemical-free microwave popcorn on page 97.

BEVERAGES

Water is an important part of a healthy diet, but should you buy bottled or filtered water, or is tap water okay? It really depends on the quality of your local water. Some water may be perfectly healthy but have a flavor you find unpleasant. It's also possible for water that tastes fine to contain contaminants. Water quality may also vary at different times of the year.

Many people assume that government regulations ensure the quality and safety of the water supply. But the regulations may not be as strict as you think and there are enforcement issues. If you are on a public water system, you are supposed to get a report every summer with details about your water quality and any contaminants that have been found in it. It's often included with your water bill. If you're a renter, you probably never see these reports. But many are posted online on the Environmental Protection Agency's Web site. Another alternative is to have your water tested by an independent laboratory. You'll want to choose a state-certified laboratory. You can find one in your area by calling the Safe Drinking Water Hotline at 800-426-4791 or visiting www.epa.gov/safewater/labs

Bottled Water

Bottled water is not necessarily any purer or better tasting than the water that runs out of your tap. Here's a guide to the types of bottled water you're likely to find on the shelves.

TAP WATER, ONLY BETTER—Some major brands of bottled water, like Dasani and Aquafina, use tap water that's charcoal-filtered and purified using reverse osmosis. In the process, trace minerals are removed, which can give the water a flat taste. Some brands (such as Dasani) add minerals back in after purification in order to improve the flavor. It's not enough minerals to make a big difference nutritionally, however.

SPRING WATER—Other brands, like Poland Spring and Deer Park, come from natural springs. This water is filtered naturally through sand and gravel and contains whatever minerals it acquires in the process. Spring water is usually tested regularly for contaminants and impurities. The mineral content of natural spring water can range from very low to high enough to have a noticeable impact on intake of certain nutrients. Spring water that has substantial mineral content is usually sold as "mineral water."

MYSTERY WATER—Brands that provide little or no information about where the water comes from or how it was processed may be nothing more than bottled tap water.

DISTILLED WATER—Purified using steam distillation, it is absolutely pure—not counting any plastic that might leach into it while it's sitting in the bottle. Because all trace minerals are also removed in the process, distilled water tastes sort of flat and is slightly more acidic than regular tap water.

SELTZER AND CLUB SODA—These are filtered or tap water with added carbonation. In some cases, sodium is also added (check the Nutrition Facts label). They may also be flavored with fruit flavors such as lime or lemon. Seltzer is naturally calorie- and sugar-free. Although the carbonation makes it slightly more acidic than regular water, drinking selzer water is not associated with any of the health issues (such as calcium loss or damage to tooth enamel) that I describe below in the section on soda. There appear to be no long-term consequences to drinking your water with bubbles if you prefer it that way.

Make Your Own Seltzer

If you drink a lot of seltzer water, you can save money and reduce waste with an environmentally friendly soda maker, such as the Soda-Stream, which carbonates tap or filtered water using a refillable CO_2 cartridge. No more recycling, no more waste, no more hauling cases of selzer water home from the store. I couldn't live without mine. Find them online at www.sodastream.com or at 1-800-763-2258.

Mineral Water

Mineral water is spring water that has a substantial amount of dissolved minerals in it. It may be still or sparkling. The amount and type of minerals give waters from various sources a distinctive taste. In some cases, they provide substantial amounts of nutrients. For example, Gerolsteiner is particularly high in calcium and magnesium, while Vichy Catalán contains a notable amount of sodium. See the table below to learn how much various mineral waters can contribute to your daily intake.

Mineral Content Per One Liter of Water

BRAND	CALCIUM	MAGNESIUM	POTASSIUM	SODIUM
Apollinaris	100 mg (10% DV)	130 mg (33% DV)	20 mg (<1% DV)	410 mg (17% DV)
Gerolsteiner	348 mg (35% DV)	108 mg (27% DV)	11 mg (<1% DV)	118 mg (5% DV)
Perrier	170 mg (17% DV)	6 mg (2% DV)	1.5 mg (<1% DV)	12 mg (<1% DV)
San Pellegrino	200 mg (20% DV)	52 mg (10% DV)	4 mg (<1% DV)	36 mg (2% DV)
Vichy Catalán	54 mg (5% DV)	9 mg (2% DV)	48 mg (1% DV)	1110 mg (46% DV)

Water Filters

One potential downside to bottled water is that the bottles themselves create an enormous amount of environmental waste. In addition, compounds can leach into the water from plastic containers, especially when stored for long periods or at high temperatures. My solution is to filter the water at home, using an inexpensive microbiological filter, and to use stainless steel reusable water bottles when I'm out and about.

If you do decide to invest in a water purification system, there are a lot of options to consider. There are units that mount on your faucet, systems that sit on the counter or under the sink, and whole-house systems that purify the water as it comes into your house. You can spend anywhere from a couple of hundred dollars to several thousand. You'll also want to match the technology to your specific concerns. For example, distillation systems do a great job removing bacteria and heavy metals but they're not so great at removing chemicals found in pesticides and herbicides. Multimedia filtration systems do a good job removing chemicals, heavy metals, and microorganisms but it can take a long time for the water to go through the filters, which can be a hassle if you're trying to filter all the water you use. On the plus side, filtration systems usually don't use any electricity.

If you're considering a purification system, it's important to know what, if anything, you're dealing with in your local water supply—because this may determine what type of system you need. If you live in an agricultural area, for example, pesticides and fertilizer runoff is a concern. If you live in an area where there is mining, there could be heavy metals in the water. If there is a lot of manufacturing or other industry close by, solvents may be a bigger problem. (See "Beverages" on page 98 for water-testing resources.)

How Much Water Do You Need to Drink?

I bet you've heard it said that you need to drink at least eight glasses of water a day in order to stay properly hydrated. Like most urban legends, the two-liter-a-day rule does have some basis in fact. The average person needs about two liters, or approximately eight glasses, of water a day to replace what is lost through normal biological functions like breathing, sweating, and urinating. But that doesn't mean that you need to drink two liters of water. In fact, hypothetically, you don't have to drink any water at all. For one thing, you can easily get a liter or liter and a half of water just from the food that you eat, especially if you eat lots of fruits and vegetables, which are up to 97 percent water. Coffee, tea, and soda also contribute toward your fluid quota. (See "Caffeine: Setting the Record Straight," page 109.)

If you're involved in sustained, strenuous exercise or spend extended periods of time in very hot or dry conditions, you'll definitely need extra fluids to stay adequately hydrated. Nursing mothers also need additional fluids. And because the thirst reflex declines with age, the elderly are at a higher risk of dehydration. But barring ill health, extremely hot or dry conditions, and intense physical activity, most people can stay well hydrated by eating a reasonably healthy diet and drinking water or other nonalcoholic beverages when they are thirsty. As a rule of thumb, if you are peeing several times a day and your urine is pale in color, you are doing fine.

Most people can stay adequately hydrated on significantly less than eight glasses of water a day.

Soda

Soda is fine as an occasional treat but as a dietary staple—which it has become, it's an unmitigated disaster. A single soda contains enough sugar to blow your sugar budget for the entire day. Soda is also quite acidic, and the combination of sugar and acid is extremely tough on tooth enamel. Finally, some flavors (usually the brown-colored ones) contain phosphates, which can increase calcium losses. When your diet contains plenty of calcium, that isn't a problem. But soda has replaced milk as the standard beverage for kids. That translates to reduced calcium intake and increased calcium losses during the critical years that we need to be accumulating enough bone density to last a lifetime. It's a perfect storm that's now leading to people being diagnosed with osteoporosis before they're even out of middle age. The increase in soda consumption is also the primary driving factor in childhood obesity—and it's going a long way toward keeping adults overweight, as well. Soda isn't really a beverage; it's liquid candy, and I'd encourage you to think of it the same way—as something to be consumed in small quantities (nothing larger than a 12-ounce can) and only once in a while.

THE QUICK AND DIRTY SECRET

Unless you're trying to gain weight, it's a good idea not to drink your calories.

Diet Drinks

Artificially sweetened sodas and noncarbonated soft drinks like Crystal Light don't have the sugar and calories of regular soda. However, the phosphates in diet soda can still lead to bone loss, especially if your diet isn't high in calcium. Diet soda also doesn't appear to be very effective in preventing weight gain. Studies show that the more diet soda you drink, the more likely you are to gain weight. (See also "Do Artificial Sweeteners Help with Weight Loss?" on page 65.) Although sipping artificially sweetened lemonade throughout the day may help you drink more water, it's also a good way to train a sweet tooth.

Artificially sweetened drinks may offer some advantages over sweetened beverages, but water is still best.

Fruit and Vitamin Waters

You'll also find drinks—both sweetened and artificially sweetened—with added vitamins, herbs, or fruit juice. Although these may sound like a healthy addition to your diet, they offer very little nutritional value. For those sweetened with sugar, the negative effects of the sugar far outweigh any small benefit. If you like the idea of getting a few extra nutrients, it's fine to choose a fortified option as your occasional soft drink. But I certainly wouldn't go out of my way to drink them for the nutritional benefits.

One Last Check Before You Check Out

We've completed our tour of the grocery store. But before you head to the checkout, take one last look at the contents of your cart. You should see a balance of wholesome foods, including plenty of fresh fruits and vegetables and other whole, unprocessed foods, and a minimum of junk. After all, you're essentially looking at your diet for the next several days. Make sure you feel good about what you see. If you see things in there that you'd probably be better off without, it's not too late to remove them! For a handy shopping list that recaps a lot of what we've talked about in Part One, see the Shopping Guide at the end of the book.

PART TWO
The 24-Hour Diet Makeover

Many books about diet and nutrition include elaborate meal plans, spelling out what you should eat throughout the day. For example, Breakfast Day One: one soft-boiled egg, one slice of whole-grain toast with half a teaspoon butter, one half grapefruit, and one cup of tea—and so on. To me, it seems sort of regimented and rigid (what do you do if you're allergic to eggs or grapefruit is out of season?). And although it might seem like a relief to turn all the decisions over to an expert, following a meal plan doesn't really teach you how to make good choices on your own.

In Part 2: The 24-Hour Diet Makeover, we'll go through a typical day, from breakfast to bedtime, and tackle all of the food and nutrition decisions that might come up—including what, when, how much and how often you should eat.

I include guidelines for calories and portion sizes, but to keep things simple, I've given recommendations for the average person, or ranges that cover the majority of people. But one size obviously won't fit all. How many calories you need depends on your age, size, and activity level. Wherever I've given ranges, the lower end of the range applies to smaller, older, and/or less active people; the higher end is for larger, younger, and/or more active people. To get a more accurate and personalized estimate of how many calories you should eat, try the online calculators at mayoclinic.com or nutritiondata.com

Although I do include suggestions for healthy meals (as well as a few sample meal plans at the end of the book), my goal is not to make all the decisions for you but rather to show you how to make healthier choices as you go through your day. As you'll see, it's not as difficult as those bite-by-bite meal plans might imply.

I'm also not going to endorse a specific diet doctrine. Diet philosophies—vegan, hunter-gatherer, Mediterranean, high-protein, low-carb, and so on—go in and out of fashion, both in the public imagination and in the hearts and minds of nutrition scientists and researchers. Each has its merits but I don't think any one of them is the single solution for every eater. Certain nutrition principles apply across the board (and those are the ones that I'll be focusing on most), but there are lots of ways to put together a healthy diet. Let's find the one that works for you.

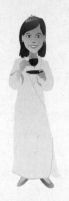

CHAPTER FOUR

Breakfast of Divas

THERE IS A lot of nutritional lore about breakfast—and, as is typical of lore, only some of it is based on actual science. I'll show you which bits of conventional wisdom you should take to heart and which you can safely ignore. Not everyone's day starts in the morning, of course. But whether you work traditional office hours or the night shift, this chapter is about how you *break* the *fast* that occurs while you sleep and recharge your batteries. I'll cover some of the common breakfast foods we reach for in the morning and tell you whether or not they are good choices, and I'll help you put together a healthy and complete breakfast customized to your own personal tastes and nutritional requirements.

COFFEE, TEA, OR CAFFEINE FREE?

The first thing many people (including me) think about when they open their eyes is getting a cup of coffee or tea. If you're one of those who can't get started in the morning without a caffeinated beverage, you'll be glad to hear that caffeine has a lot of positive health benefits and, despite what you may have heard, relatively few drawbacks. Caffeine is a mild stimulant that affects the brain and central nervous system. It makes you more alert and boosts your ability to concentrate. Caffeine doesn't make you any smarter but a little caffeine can help you do better on tests. It also won't make you any more sober, but (assuming you *are* sober) it can enhance your driving skills. Regular caffeine consumption seems to have a protective effect on the central nervous system as well, reducing your risk of Alzheimer's and Parkinson's.

Caffeine also enhances athletic performance. In fact, up until recently, caffeine was considered a performance-enhancing drug by the International Olympic Committee and athletes had to keep their intake of caffeinated beverages fairly low to pass their drug screens. Unlike most performance-enhancing drugs, you can safely try this one at home.

THE QUICK AND DIRTY SECRET

Have a caffeinated beverage one hour before your workout and you may be able to go a bit faster, stronger, and longer.

Downsides of Caffeine

Some people find that too much caffeine makes them jittery, anxious, or disrupts their sleep. How many cups of coffee it takes to make *your* hair stand on end, or how late in the day you can drink a cup of coffee without staring at the ceiling all night, is subject to a high degree of individual variation.

If you drink coffee or other caffeinated beverages regularly, you're much less likely to experience negative side effects from caffeine. That's because caffeine is highly habituating. Your brain gets used to having it around—and notices if it suddenly disappears. The biggest problem with being habituated to caffeine is that you might feel a little sleepy or get a headache if you suddenly swear it off. These withdrawal symptoms are harmless and usually last only a few days. (Medical researchers have discovered that a lot of post-surgical headaches are actually due to caffeine withdrawal and can be prevented by adding a bit of caffeine to the intravenous fluids administered during recovery!) If for some reason you decide you want to stop consuming caffeine, you can make it easier on yourself by tapering your consumption off over the course of a couple of weeks.

LET'S TAKE A CLOSER LOOK

Caffeine: Setting the Record Straight

Many of the negative things you've heard about caffeine are actually myths.

Caffeine does not increase pain, tenderness, or benign lumps in the breast. Although there are persistent rumors to this effect, study after study has found no reliable correlation between caffeine consumption and breast pain. Some women find that swearing off caffeine gives them relief from painful symptoms. But if eliminating caffeine doesn't help you, there's no reason not to resume drinking it if you choose. And if you don't have breast pain or lumps, caffeine will not increase your risk of developing them.

Caffeine does not weaken your bones. It's true that when you take in more caffeine you tend to lose more calcium in your urine. However, your body is pretty smart. It can compensate for these losses by increasing the amount of calcium that it absorbs from the foods you eat. As long as your diet contains enough calcium, caffeine consumption has little or no long-term effect on bone health.

Caffeinated beverages are not dehydrating. Caffeine is a diuretic, meaning that it increases urine output, but when you drink caffeinated beverages, you're still taking in more fluids than you lose. If you don't drink caffeinated beverages regularly, drinking a cup of coffee ends up being the equivalent of drinking about two-thirds of a cup of water. In other words, drinking coffee and tea will hydrate you—just not quite as efficiently as water will. However, if you regularly drink caffeinated beverages, research demonstrates that the diuretic effects are almost negligible. Your body retains the same amount of fluid from a cup of coffee or tea as it does from a cup of water. (Caffeine pills, on the other hand, don't contain any fluids and can be dehydrating.)

Caffeine is not bad for your heart. Certain studies have found that drinking unfiltered coffee—such as French press or percolated coffee—elevates cholesterol in some men. Despite this, coffee drinkers are no more likely to develop heart disease. And although caffeinated coffee can temporarily increase your heart rate a bit, it does not cause arrhythmia, or irregular heartbeat.

A Few Reasons to Avoid Caffeine

Most people tolerate caffeine just fine but there are a few reasons you might choose not to consume it. People who are very sensitive to stimulants are usually better off avoiding caffeine altogether. In addition, caffeine does appear to negatively affect the growth and development of babies in the womb, so pregnant women are advised to limit their intake.

Although caffeine doesn't cause heart disease, it can temporarily increase your heart rate and your blood pressure. So people who already have heart problems and who are sensitive to caffeine may want to avoid it. Even if there's only a small possibility that a jolt of caffeine will trigger a problem, many feel it's just not worth the risk! For everyone else, consuming a moderate amount of caffeine appears to have some benefits and limited disadvantages, so stop worrying and enjoy your morning cup of coffee and tea.

How Much Caffeine Is Healthy?

A cup of coffee or a couple of cups of black tea every day is enough to get some positive benefit. The protective effects really start piling up when you drink three or four cups of coffee a day or the equivalent. People who drink seven or eight cups a day may get even a little more benefit but also have a higher risk of ill effects. And more than that is not advisable.

To maximize the benefits without overdoing it, limit your daily caffeine consumption to 600–800 milligrams, or the equivalent of 3–4 cups of regular coffee.

How Much Caffeine Is in It?

Coca-cola (12 ounce can) 35 mg
Mountain Dew (12 ounce can) 54 mg
Ginger Ale (12 ounce can) 0 mg
Regular strength coffee (12 ounces) 150–200 mg
Decaf coffee (12 ounces) 15 mg
Espresso (1 ounce) 70 mg
Latte (16 ounces) 150 mg
Black tea (8 ounces) 40–60 mg
Snapple Unsweetened Iced Tea (16 ounces) 18 mg
Green tea (8 ounces) 20–40 mg
White tea (8 ounces) 15–20 mg
Herbal tea (8 ounces) 0 mg
Coffee liqueur (1 ounce) 9 mg

Which Is Better: Coffee or Tea?

As for whether to get your caffeine from coffee or tea, each contains unique active compounds and each is associated with different health benefits. People who drink coffee every day have a significantly lower risk of diabetes, Parkinson's, colon cancer, gallstones, and Alzheimer's disease. Drinking black or green tea can reduce your risk of heart disease, stroke, and cancer. Green tea has also been linked to reduced risk of gum disease and osteoporosis. In terms of their health benefits, I don't think a clear case can be made for one over the other. Drink whichever you prefer—or all of the above! Now that you've got both eyes open, it's time to think about breakfast.

Will You Burn More Fat if You Exercise Before Breakfast?

Some people claim that you'll burn more fat or calories if you exercise before breakfast. How many *calories* you burn during exercise mostly depends on how hard and long you exercise, not how long it's been since you've eaten. But there is some research showing that if you exercise on an empty stomach you will burn more *fat* than if you did the same exercise later in the day.

Why? Your body stores energy (or calories) in a variety of formats and places in your body. You store a little bit in your blood, a little bit in your muscles, some in your liver, and the rest you store as body fat. It's a little like storing your money in a number of different places. You probably have some in your wallet, possibly some more in your dresser drawer, some in a checking account, and maybe the rest is in a money-market account. Which account you withdraw funds from will probably depend on how much you need and how fast you need it.

Similarly, what type of fuel you burn during exercise depends in part on the balances available in your various fuel storage accounts. In the morning, your blood, muscle, and liver "accounts" are going to be at their lowest, because your body will have been drawing on them to pay for metabolic activities during the ten or twelve hours since you had your last meal. So, if you exercise first thing in the morning, before you've refilled those energy accounts by eating some breakfast, you're going to have to tap into those fat stores that much sooner.

But does this really change how much body fat you will lose in the long run? Not really. Just like with your money, regardless of which account you withdraw from, you're still spending the same amount. If you spend more than you deposit, your net worth goes down. And when you burn more calories than you take in, you're going to lose body fat.

Exercising on an empty stomach may increase the amount of body fat you burn *during* exercise. But your body alternately makes and burns body fat all day long, transferring fuel in and out of its various accounts. So, you might burn a bit more fat while you're exercising on an empty stomach but then burn a bit less fat later in the day. Over the long term, the amount of fat you have in your body depends mostly on how many calories you take in versus how many calories you burn and not when you burn them.

When you get right down to it, the most effective workout is the one you actually show up for on a regular basis. If working out first thing in the morning fits your schedule better, then an early morning workout is probably going to be more effective for you.

On the other hand, if you find that you get a better workout at the end of the day when you've got some steam to blow off, then that's probably the best time of day for you to exercise. Or, maybe you have a workout partner who is only available after work. Having a date to meet someone at the gym or track might make you much more likely to follow through with your exercise plans.

THE QUICK AND DIRTY SECRET

The best time to exercise is when it's convenient and enjoyable for you.

WHEN TO EAT BREAKFAST

Some people wake up hungry; others are ready for breakfast within an hour or so; some may not feel hungry until they've been up for several hours. A lot depends on the timing and size of the previous night's dinner as well as your exercise routine and schedule, so I'm willing to be flexible about the timing of your first meal—but not about the quality. The problem with delaying breakfast is that your ability to make healthy choices may be limited once your day is underway. Instead of scrambled eggs, or yogurt and fruit, or a bowl of oatmeal you end up eating a donut or two at the staff meeting, or heading for the office vending machine or the closest drive-thru. I'll make a deal with you: You don't have to eat breakfast at the crack of dawn, but you do need to have a plan for a healthy meal—and a schedule that will allow you to take a break when you do get hungry.

Important Note: If you have diabetes, hypoglycemia, are pregnant, or have other health conditions, it may be particularly important to stick to a regular meal schedule. Please check with your health professional before departing from your prescribed eating plan.

Breakfast and Weight Control

People who skip breakfast are more likely to be overweight. Now, why would skipping breakfast make you fat? Shouldn't skipping meals actually lead to weight loss? One popular theory is that eating breakfast gives a little bump to your metabolism, which slows slightly during sleep. If you skip breakfast, the theory goes, your metabolism stays sluggish until you eat lunch. According to this idea, the earlier you eat breakfast, the more calories you'll burn throughout the day. But before you reset your alarm clock, you should know that there is little hard evidence that the timing of your first meal has any *meaningful* effect on your total calorie burning for the day. (I'll talk more about the effect of meal timing on your metabolism in the next chapter.)

The second explanation for why people who skip breakfast are more likely to be overweight is that they end up getting overly hungry and making poor choices later in the day. They either overcompensate by eating too much at lunch, or they grab whatever is around when hunger hits and end up eating junk food instead of a more nutritious breakfast. That's a little more plausible than the metabolism theory. If you are having trouble managing your weight and you don't eat breakfast regularly, it's definitely worth seeing whether getting into a regular breakfast routine helps move you closer to your goal. But there's nothing to say that postponing that first meal of the day must *inevitably* lead to overeating or unhealthy food choices. That's the beauty of being grown-ups: We do have some control over these things.

THE QUICK AND DIRTY SECRET

Skipping breakfast won't trash your metabolism but it may lead to poor choices later in the day.

How Late Is Too Late to Eat Breakfast?

It's OK to wait until you're hungry before eating breakfast but waiting until you're famished often leads to poor food choices—both in terms of quality and quantity. Plan your day so that you can eat breakfast before you have reached that point. If you find yourself overeating later in the day, it's an indication that you may have delayed your first meal too long. Hunger, by the way, can announce itself in a number of ways. You may or may not experience the sensation of having an empty stomach. If you are feeling sleepy, unfocused, or have a headache and it's been more than four hours since your last meal, it may be that you are hungry. Masking these symptoms with caffeine is not an acceptable substitute for a nutritious meal.

WHAT TO EAT FOR BREAKFAST

Many traditional breakfast foods, such as cereal, bread, and fruit, are mostly carbohydrates—and these foods serve a valuable function at breakfast. By morning, it's probably been eight to twelve hours since your last meal and your body's energy reserves have been depleted. Carbohydrates will rapidly replenish the energy stores that fuel your brain and muscles. But a ride on the blood-sugar roller coaster is not what we're after. Sugary breakfast cereals and pastries—even the organic ones!—can send blood sugar soaring, and then crashing, which can make you feel dizzy, weak, and just generally not well. Instead, choose whole fruit (rather than juice) and whole-grain breads and cereals that are low in sugar and high in fiber. (Remember the Rule of Five on page 57.) These types of carbohydrates are digested more slowly and aren't as likely to result in an unpleasant energy crash an hour after breakfast. Studies also show that people who eat more fiber tend to be leaner and are less likely to gain weight over time.

Don't Gorge on Granola

Despite its healthy reputation, granola is often very high in sugar and calories. A better choice is muesli, which contains all the whole grains, nuts, and fruit of granola without the extra sugar and oil. Either way, be sure to check the serving size on the Nutrition Facts label. A serving of granola or muesli is usually a third to half as big as a serving of other cereals.

What's the Difference Between Soluble and Insoluble Fiber?

If you stirred some soluble fiber into hot water, it would dissolve. In your stomach, the soluble fiber you've eaten dissolves in water from your food and/or digestive juices and makes a viscous liquid or gel. This gel can trap certain food components and make them less available for absorption.

In particular, soluble fiber interferes somewhat with the absorption of fats and sugars. Now, before you get too excited about this, let me clarify that soluble fiber doesn't keep you from absorbing calories from foods high in fat and sugar—at least, not in any meaningful way.

But its fat-binding action can help reduce cholesterol. And by slowing down the absorption of sugar, fiber helps keep blood sugar levels steadier—which is helpful for managing and preventing diabetes.

If you stir some insoluble fiber into hot water, it won't dissolve. As soon as you stop stirring, it'll just sink to the bottom. It will, however, soak up a bunch of the water and puff up, the way a dry sponge expands as it soaks up water. Now imagine this puffed-up sponge moving through your intestines and you'll begin to get an idea what insoluble fiber does for you. Insoluble fiber is a very effective treatment and preventive for constipation and other digestive disorders like diverticulosis and irritable bowel syndrome.

Important Note: In some cases, people with acute digestive problems are advised to reduce the amount of fiber in their diet—at least temporarily, until things calm down. If you're being treated by a physician, be sure to follow his or her recommendations about your diet.

Which Type of Fiber Should You Eat?

Most foods contain a mixture of soluble and insoluble fiber. The inside of apples, for example, provides soluble fiber and the skins contain mostly insoluble fiber. The dietary recommendations for fiber are 25 grams per day for women and 38 grams per day for men. There are no guidelines for how much of that should be soluble or insoluble. In the typical diet, about three-quarters of the fiber is insoluble and one quarter is soluble. I think that reflects the fact that we tend to eat a lot of grain-based foods and not enough fruits and vegetables.

If you're particularly concerned with keeping your blood sugar steady or your cholesterol down, you might want to focus on eating more legumes and oats, which are good sources of soluble fiber. If digestive health or constipation is a problem, you might want to emphasize foods that contain a lot of insoluble fiber, such as flaxseed, wheat, corn, and rice bran. But chances are you could do with more of *both* kinds of fiber. Most people get less than half the recommended amount.

Make Old-fashioned Oats as Quick as Instant

If you prefer the very soft texture of instant oats to the nubbier, chewier texture of regular rolled oats, this tip isn't for you. But if the main attraction of instant oats is the quick preparation time, here's how to make old-fashioned oats almost as quickly: Place one-half cup regular (old-fashioned) rolled oats and one cup water into a microwave-safe bowl, along with a pinch of salt, if desired. (If you like your oatmeal a little soupier, use one-third cup oats.) Cover bowl with a lid or inverted plate and microwave on high for two-and-a-half to three minutes. Voila! In the time it takes to wait for the kettle to boil to make instant, you can enjoy all hearty goodness of old-fashioned oatmeal.

☞ **See also my recipes for Apple Pie Oatmeal and Warm Weather Oats in the recipe section that begins on page 197.**

Breakfast Should Also Include Protein

Although carbohydrates are a good way to refuel, an all-carbohydrate breakfast (such as a piece of toast and glass of juice) is not ideal. You also want some slower-burning protein, which will keep your energy up and your hunger at bay until your next meal. A lot of people tend to skimp on protein at breakfast—especially when time is tight. If you find yourself getting hungry an hour or two after breakfast, it's a sign that you may need to pump up the protein.

How Much Protein Do You Need?

Try to include at least 15 grams of protein in your morning meal. More is okay, too. (I'll be talking a lot more about protein—including how much you need over the course of a typical day—in the next chapter.) As you'll see in the table on page 126, a container of yogurt or a splash of milk on your cereal is not quite enough to get the job done. Here are some easy ways to add more protein to typical carb-heavy breakfasts:

Instead of butter or jam, top your toast or bagel with peanut butter, cheese, or smoked fish.

Sprinkle a small handful of chopped nuts on your cereal or yogurt.

Blend a chunk of tofu into your smoothie.

THE QUICK AND DIRTY SECRET

Breakfasts that are high in protein keep you satisfied longer. Aim for at least 15 grams of protein at breakfast.

Eggs: Protein Power or Cholesterol Crisis?

Eggs are the classic breakfast protein, of course, but many people avoid or limit them (or eat only the whites) because of cholesterol concerns. Our parents and grandparents were taught that high blood cholesterol (which is one of several risk factors for heart disease) was caused by eating foods that are high in cholesterol. Now we know better. About 10 percent of the population has an exaggerated response to cholesterol in foods. Unless you're one of those people, however, the cholesterol in the *foods* you eat has very little effect on the amount of cholesterol in your *blood*. The vast majority of people can eat a couple eggs a day without raising their cholesterol levels or increasing their risk of heart disease. If you have high cholesterol or heart disease, it's important to consult with your doctor or nutritionist about what's right for you. Otherwise, the cholesterol in eggs is one of those things you can stop worrying about!

THE QUICK AND DIRTY SECRET

Stop throwing away your egg yolks! Not only is the cholesterol unlikely to cause a problem, but the yolks are where a lot of the nutrients (like vitamins D and E) are found.

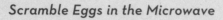

Scramble Eggs in the Microwave

For a quick, nutritious breakfast with no pots or pans to clean, try scrambling your eggs in the microwave. To begin, crack an egg or two into a glass bowl. Whisk the eggs with a fork or whisk until the yolks and whites are blended. Add a dash of salt and pepper (and a sprinkle of grated cheese if you like) and pop in the microwave for thirty seconds. Give the eggs a stir and return them to the microwave. If the eggs are almost done after the first thirty seconds, give them another fifteen seconds. If they are still fairly runny after that, microwave for another thirty seconds.

Breakfast Meats

If you're looking for a way to add more protein to your breakfast, meat would seem to be an obvious answer (for nonvegetarians, anyway). But traditional breakfast meats like bacon, ham, and sausage are usually made with nitrites, which are best avoided. (See the discussion on nitrites on page 38.) Even nitrite-free products tend to be high in fat and sodium. And as you can see in the tables on pages 126–127, there are plenty of other ways to get protein at breakfast.

Although they are okay to have every once in a while, I don't recommend eating bacon or sausage on a daily basis. And when you do have bacon, be sure to cook it slowly over low heat (or in the microwave) and be very careful not to burn it. Cooking bacon over high heat or until it's extra crisp accelerates the conversion of nitrites into harmful nitrosamines. For the same reason, avoid ordering bacon extra-crisp in restaurants.

Is Turkey Bacon Really Healthier?

A lot of people assume that turkey bacon is inherently healthier than bacon from pork. But cold cuts, bacon, and sausages made from turkey or chicken can contain just as much fat and sodium as their traditional counterparts. They're also just as likely to be made with nitrites. And regardless of what kind of meat they're made from, low-fat versions of these foods are usually even higher in sodium than the regular-fat varieties. Before opting for these alternatives, check the Nutrition Facts labels and ingredients lists to be sure that they are, indeed, healthier options.

Smoothies

Made with the right ingredients, smoothies can make a nutritious breakfast (they can also make a good snack or post-workout meal). But if you're not careful, a smoothie can easily turn into a sugar-loaded calorie bomb. Here's how to make a smoothie that's both good and good for you.

STEP 1: CHOOSE A BASE—First, you need some sort of liquid or semiliquid base. You can use milk or a nondairy alternative such as soymilk—but if you use soy or another nondairy milk, remember that even the plain, unsweetened ones can have a lot of added sugar. As I suggested in chapter 1, try to find a brand that has no more than 12 grams of sugar per eight-ounce serving. Even better, use plain yogurt as the base of your smoothie and you'll get the additional benefits of the beneficial bacteria it contains. Avoid using fruit juice as the base for your smoothie. My biggest gripe with smoothies from commercial juice bars is that they're usually made with a lot of fruit juice and, as a result, are very high in sugar and calories. Put about one cup of base into the jar of your blender.

STEP 2: ADD FRUIT—Fruit adds sweetness to your smoothie as well as fiber and other nutrients. If you use frozen fruit, it will also make your smoothie thick and frosty, sort of like a milkshake. Frozen bananas are great for this because they contain pectin, a sort of fiber that makes the smoothie extra creamy-tasting. Whenever you have bananas that are getting a little too ripe, toss them in the freezer to use for smoothies. (Be sure to peel your bananas *before* freezing them.) Frozen strawberries are also terrific in smoothies, as are peaches and mangoes. Blueberries and raspberries, although they are quite nutritious, tend to be a little gritty in smoothies. Add about one serving of fruit to the blender. If you prefer to use fresh, unfrozen fruit, add a couple of ice cubes as well.

STEP 3: ADD PROTEIN—A cup of milk, soymilk, or yogurt contains about ten grams of protein (other nondairy milks contain much less). To make the smoothie a bit more substantial, add some extra protein. Some people like to use protein powders for this but I think its preferable to get your nutrition from foods rather than supplements whenever possible. You can boost the protein content of your smoothie by adding a chunk of tofu or a couple of tablespoons of peanut butter or other nut butter. Peanut butter goes particularly well in smoothies that contain bananas. I don't recommend adding raw egg to your smoothie, Rocky-style. Not only is there a slight danger of salmonella poisoning with uncooked eggs, but your body absorbs the protein in eggs much better when they're cooked.

STEP 4: BLEND YOUR SMOOTHIE—Whiz everything in the blender on high until it's completely blended. If your smoothie is too thick, you may be using too much frozen fruit or too many ice cubes. Thin it by adding a bit of water or even a splash of green tea or coffee. Coffee goes particularly well in smoothies made with banana, nut butter, and/or cocoa powder. Green tea is a great match for a strawberry or peaches. Both tea and coffee add beneficial antioxidants, not to mention caffeine, which has its own benefits. (You can even use coffee or green tea as part of the liquid in step one.) If your smoothie isn't sweet enough for your taste, you can add a bit of honey or maple syrup, but keep in mind that even natural sweeteners like honey and maple syrup should be consumed in moderation. You could also use a sugar-free sweetener like stevia.

OPTIONAL EXTRAS—You can dress up your smoothie with all kinds of extras.

Flaxseeds Add two tablespoons of flaxseeds to add some extra fiber, protein, and a nice helping of omega-3 fatty acids. **Quick Tip:** Flaxseed contains a lot of soluble fiber, which tends to absorb liquid and form a gel. That's great when it happens in your body; not so great when it happens in your glass. If you're not going to be drinking your smoothie within twenty minutes or so, you might want to leave the flax out.

Cocoa Powder It's jam-packed with flavanols—the compounds that make chocolate so good for you. But unlike chocolate, it's low in calories, contains no sugar, and is virtually fat-free. Add a tablespoon of cocoa powder for a heart-healthy boost. Cocoa powder tastes good in smoothies made with bananas and/or nut butter. **Quick Tip:** If it's the health benefits of cocoa you're after, avoid Dutch-processed or alkalized cocoa powder, which has less than half the flavanol content of regular cocoa powder.

Raw Spinach A lot of people like to throw in a handful of raw spinach or other leafy greens. Although it turns your smoothie a bright, virtuous-looking green color, you can't really taste them and it's a great way to sneak another serving of vegetables into your day. Greens go well with strawberry- or peach-flavored smoothies. **Quick Tip:** Greens, especially spinach, contain oxalates, which are compounds that can interfere with your ability to absorb calcium. If the milk or yogurt in your smoothie is your primary source of calcium, you might want to save the greens and have them at a different meal.

THE REALITY CHECK—Finally, just because it's packed with nutrition and maybe even spinach, doesn't mean that the calories in that smoothie don't count. Make sure that you have a realistic grip on how many calories your smoothie contains so that you know how it fits into your overall diet plan. Here's a chart of common smoothie ingredients that you can use to see how your favorite smoothie adds up.

Smoothie Calculator

SMOOTHIE INGREDIENT	FIBER (G)	CALORIES	PROTEIN (G)
1 cup 2% milk	0	122	8
1 cup soymilk	2	110	9
1 cup lowfat yogurt	0	154	13
1 medium banana	3	105	1
3/4 cup frozen strawberries	2	38	1
3/4 cup frozen peaches	2	60	1
2 ounces tofu	1	48	5
2 tablespoons peanut butter	2	180	7
2 tablespoons flaxseed	6	110	4
1 tablespoon cocoa powder	2	12	1
1 cup spinach	1	7	1
1 teaspoon honey	0	20	0
1 teaspoon maple syrup	0	13	0

Think Outside the Cereal Box

Finally, don't be afraid to think outside the cereal box. Being a bit more flexible about what you consider to be breakfast fare can open up a lot of nutritious options. For example, there's no reason why you can't eat vegetables for breakfast! (See my recipe for Leftover Vegetable Frittata on page 200.) Fish is also a terrific way to get protein at breakfast, and offers a nutritional bonus in the form of omega-3 fats. You can fold leftover fish into an omelet or enjoy smoked fish on a whole-grain bagel or crackers with a big slice of ripe tomato. Or roll scrambled eggs, beans, and cheese into a tortilla for a Breakfast Burrito (recipe on page 201).

Here are some traditional breakfast foods from other countries to jump-start your imagination:

Israel: Salad of feta cheese, watermelon, and cucumber
Japan: Miso soup with tofu
Scandinavia: Pickled herring on rye crisps
Jamaica: Sardines and ripe plantains
India: Spiced lentils and rice

HOW MUCH TO EAT FOR BREAKFAST

"Eat breakfast like a king, lunch like a prince, and supper like a pauper," is an oft-repeated—but rarely followed—piece of dietary advice. Eating a large breakfast might be good advice if people really did taper off the size of their meals as they went through the day. In reality, however, people who eat very large breakfasts often end up eating more calories over the course of a day than those who eat smaller breakfasts.

As a general rule, plan to eat between 25 and 30 percent of the day's calories between the time you wake up and lunchtime. For most people, that's between 400 and 700 calories. (The lower end of the range is for those who are smaller, older, and/or less active; the higher end of the range is for people who are larger, younger, and/or more active.)

THE QUICK AND DIRTY SECRET

Eat at least a quarter of your daily calories before lunchtime.

Healthy Breakfasts

MENU	CALORIES (APPROX.)	FIBER (G)	PROTEIN (G)
Oatmeal with chopped apples and walnuts, latte	400	6	16
Breakfast Burrito (recipe on page 201), fruit salad	500	6	23
Smoothie with soymilk, banana, and almond butter; Fruit and Nut bar (recipe on page 206)	600	12	25
Omelet (3 eggs) with smoked salmon, tomato, spinach, and cream cheese; 2 pieces whole-grain toast with butter	700	10	32

I've given some examples of healthy breakfasts in the table above. The following table shows you nutritional values for common breakfast foods so you can also build your own. If you don't have a big appetite in the morning, you can divide breakfast into two smaller meals and have the second one as a midmorning snack. I'll have much more to say about the pros and cons of snacking in chapter 6.

Nutrition Guide to Breakfast Foods

FOOD (TYPICAL SERVING)	CALORIES	FIBER (G)	PROTEIN (G)
2 eggs	160	0	12
1 cup 2% milk	122	0	8
1 skim latte (tall)	100	0	10
1 cup soy milk	110	3	10
1 cup rice milk	100	0	1
1 cup plain yogurt	150	0	11
1/2 cup cottage cheese	85	0	14

FOOD (TYPICAL SERVING)	CALORIES	FIBER (G)	PROTEIN (G)
1 small handful nuts	185	2	5
2 tablespoons cream cheese	60	0	2
2 tablespoons nut butter	180	2	8
1 ounce smoked salmon	100	0	5
1 ounce cheese	110	0	8
2 sausage link	129	0	9
2 strips bacon	85	0	6
3 slices Canadian bacon	87	0	11
1 slice tofu (⅕ package)	66	1	7
1 bowl oatmeal	166	4	6
1 piece whole wheat toast	76	2	4
1 pat butter	36	0	0
1 cup fruit	75	3	1
½ cup fruit juice	65	0	1
½ cup cooked vegetables	35	3	0

Check the Nutrition Facts label for serving size and nutrition information for your favorite ready-to-eat cereal.

BREAKFAST ON THE FLY

No doubt there will also be times when you find yourself at a restaurant, coffee shop, or even a fast-food or convenience store for breakfast. Here are some pointers on what to choose and what to avoid when you're on the road.

DINER/PANCAKE HOUSE—Avoid the waffles, pancakes, and French toast, which are low in fiber and topped with high-sugar syrups.

Instead, go for more protein and order eggs or a vegetable-stuffed omelet. Skip the hash browns and grits, which are heavy with oil, and stick to whole-grain toast.

BAKERY/COFFEE SHOP—Pass on the oversized muffins; the healthy-sounding bran muffins are often loaded with oil and the low-fat options are usually quite high in sugar. Go for the egg-and-veggie breakfast wrap or a whole-grain bagel with smoked salmon.

FAST FOOD—Skip the biscuits and croissants, which are high in calories and usually loaded with trans fats. Have an egg sandwich on an English muffin or go for the fruit and yogurt parfait.

Healthy Breakfast on the Go

CHOOSE	AVOID
English muffins	biscuits
wraps	croissants
oatmeal	grits
whole-grain toast	hash browns
fruit	juice
eggs	waffles
yogurt	pancakes
salmon	bacon
cheese	sausage

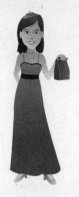

CHAPTER FIVE

Power Lunch

UNLESS YOU WORK at home, chances are good that you'll be at the office, school, or somewhere in transit when lunchtime rolls around. That can make healthy eating a bit of a challenge. In this chapter, I have some tips on what to pack for lunch. And for those times when brown-bagging isn't an option, I've also put together a survival guide for carry-out, fast-food, and casual restaurants.

The best way to avoid nutritional missteps is to bring your own lunch from home. It's also a good way to keep a few more of those hard-earned dollars in your pocket. When you make your own lunch, you control the ingredients and the portion sizes. More importantly, you have the opportunity to decide what you're going to eat ahead of time—not when you're starving.

When you wait until your stomach is growling before you start to think about what's for lunch, the outcome is fairly predictable. Good intentions fade, willpower wilts, and the next thing you know you're polishing off a greasy mountain of nachos and melted "cheez" instead of the crisp, nutritious garden salad you might have chosen under less duress. Setting aside a few minutes in the morning—or even the night before—to put together your lunch vastly increases the chances that you'll make it through the day with your healthy resolutions intact.

WHAT TO EAT FOR LUNCH

Lunch should always include at least one serving of protein such as deli-sliced turkey or roast beef, a piece of chicken or fish left over from dinner the night before, a scoop of chicken, egg, tofu, or tuna salad, a bowl of bean soup, or a handful of nuts or some nut butter. Meals that are high in protein tend to keep you satisfied for longer—and that can be helpful for those who are trying to watch their calories. Your body also needs protein for its ongoing maintenance and repair. Getting more protein will also help you recover faster from exercise and build more lean muscle.

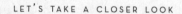

LET'S TAKE A CLOSER LOOK

Do High Protein Diets Speed Up Your Metabolism?

Eating more protein has been shown to cause your body to burn more calories, but the way these studies are reported in the press can lead to misunderstandings. For instance, researchers may be quoted as saying that high-protein meals "significantly" improve fat metabolism. When most of us hear that something made a *significant* difference, we understand that to mean that the difference was *meaningful*—because that's the way we use this word in regular life. But when statisticians say that a finding was "significant," they're only saying they're 95 percent sure that it wasn't just due to chance or random variation. In other words, an effect may be statistically significant without being terribly meaningful in the real world. So, although it may technically be true that eating more protein will cause you to burn more calories, it might take a year or two for those extra calories to add up to just one pound of weight loss. Still, every little bit counts.

How Much Protein Should You Eat?

The Institute of Medicine recommends that protein make up 10 to 35 percent of your calories—which is a pretty wide spread. The lower end of the range represents the amount you need to keep your body functioning properly. To take maximum advantage of the fat-burning, appetite-regulating, and muscle-building effects of protein, you'd want to shoot for the upper end of that range. To estimate your *maximum* recommended protein intake, figure one gram of protein for every pound you weigh. Divide that number by three to get the recommended minimum. For example, if you weigh 150 pounds, 150 grams of protein is the high end of the recommended range; 50 grams per day is the recommended minimum.

However, it's really not necessary to tote up every gram of protein you eat or to eat exactly the same amount of protein every day. Most people find it easier—and just as effective—to keep track of protein servings. To meet the minimum protein requirement, the average size person needs three to five servings of protein foods a day. Ten to twelve servings per day will bring you closer to the upper end of the range. I don't believe there's much to be gained from going any higher than that. (The Serving Size Guide at the end of the book has examples of serving sizes for different types of protein foods.)

Your body will get the most benefit from the protein you eat if you spread it throughout the day rather than eat it all at once, and that's why I recommend that every meal and snack include at least some protein. Of course, eating additional calories can lead to weight gain—even if those calories are protein. So, if you decide to step up your protein intake and you don't want to gain weight, you'll need to cut back somewhere else. If you eat a lot of sweets, junk food, or drink sweetened beverages, they should be first on the chopping block, of course. Beyond that, I suggest you offset any increase in protein foods with a proportionate decrease in starches and grain-based foods. For example, have a larger serving of tuna salad but have it on a bed of greens rather than a roll.

☛ TRY MY RECIPE FOR CURRIED TUNA SALAD, PAGE 205

Don't Forget Vegetables

Lunch should also include a serving or two of vegetables. After all, your goal is to eat at least five servings of vegetables per day. You'll have a better shot at making that target if you try to work some vegetables into most of your meals and snacks. But please don't point to that lone leaf of lettuce or that sliver of tomato on your sandwich and try to pass that off as a serving of vegetables. If you're having a sandwich, stack it up with a good half inch or so of lettuce—or, even better, spinach leaves. *That's* a serving. Or, add chopped or shredded raw vegetables (bell peppers, celery, cabbage, carrots, zucchini, etc.) to your tuna or chicken salad. The Serving Size Guide at the back of the book has more on what counts as a serving of vegetables.

☛ SEE MY RECIPE FOR TOFU SALAD WITH NUTRITIONAL
   YEAST ON PAGE 203

There's no law that says your lunch must be between two pieces of bread, either. You can roll sliced turkey, cheese, and a smear of guacamole in large Bibb lettuce leaves instead of tortillas. Stuff tuna, egg, or tofu salad into a bell pepper or beefsteak tomato instead of a roll. Or, arrange grilled chicken or fish over a mound of salad greens. Bring salad dressing in a separate container and add it right before you eat it so that you're not facing a bowl of soggy, wilted greens. If you have access to a refrigerator, consider keeping a bottle of salad dressing there.

Bread Is Optional

It's also fine to include some bread or other starch at lunchtime but it's not nutritionally necessary. In fact, if you're looking for places to trim calories, these are the ones to cut first. Compared with protein foods and vegetables, bread offers the least in the way of nutrition. And as far as keeping hunger at bay, you'll get a lot more staying power out of an extra serving of protein and/or vegetables than you will from a serving of bread. If you do have bread or grains with lunch, whole grain is your best choice.

LET'S TAKE A CLOSER LOOK

Is It Okay to Combine Protein and Starch?

There is an old but persistent idea that combining certain types of foods at the same meal is bad for your digestion. There are several variations on this theme but the most common one is that proteins and starches should never be eaten together. It's often explained like this: Starches require an alkaline environment for digestion; proteins, on the other hand, require an acidic environment for proper digestion. When you eat these foods at the same time, the digestive system, pulled into two opposite directions, supposedly stalls. Food allegedly gets "stuck" in your system, where the carbohydrates ferment and the proteins putrefy or rot.

When this theory was first put forward at the end of the nineteenth century, we didn't completely understand how the human digestive system worked. These days, we have a pretty solid understanding of how food gets digested and we can say for sure that this idea is completely false. Nonetheless, food-combination myths persist.

How Digestion Works Your digestive system is a little like a car wash. When you drive your car through the car wash, a sequence of different chemicals squirts out of a series of nozzles, aimed at various parts of your car. But your whole car goes through the entire car wash together. Similarly, everything you eat passes through your entire digestive system and the trip is pretty much the same, no matter what kind or combination of food you eat.

After you chew and swallow your food, it is treated to an acid bath in the stomach, which serves various purposes. First, the acid kills bacteria and other pathogens that could otherwise make you sick. Second, stomach acid begins to break down any proteins and prepare them for later phases of digestion. All foods, even starches and fruits, provoke this acid response in the stomach.

Next stop in the digestive car wash is the small intestine. Here the stomach acid is neutralized by pancreatic juices, which allows a variety of enzymes to go to work. (Most enzymes don't work too well in acidic environments.) There are enzymes that digest protein, enzymes that digest carbohydrates, and enzymes that digest fat. But the full array of enzymes is produced every time, no matter what you eat.

In other words, not only is your digestive system *capable* of digesting a combination of protein and carbohydrates, but it appears that this is the default setting. And when you think about it, it wouldn't make sense for the body to be designed to digest proteins separately from carbohydrates. Most foods that we would identify as starches contain protein. For example, about 14 percent of the calories in spaghetti are from protein. Rice and potatoes contain about 8 percent of calories from protein and wheat bread contains about 16 percent of calories from protein. On the flip side, beans and legumes—foods which supply much of the world's protein needs—contain roughly as much carbohydrate as they do protein.

THE QUICK AND DIRTY SECRET

There is no physiological or biochemical reason to avoid combining proteins and starches. In fact, adding a little protein and/or fat when you eat carbohydrates will help smooth out the rise in blood sugar that happens when you eat carbs by themselves.

A Hot Lunch

Sometimes it's nice to have a hot meal in the middle of the day. Frozen entrees, dehydrated soup mixes, and other ready-to-eat meals can also be convenient at lunchtime—and healthy options do exist.

See chapter 3 for my tips on spotting the good ones. But don't overlook what's already in the fridge. Pack up a serving of last night's dinner to reheat for lunch or get creative and reconfigure those leftovers into interesting new guises. For example, toss a cup of cooked pasta (such as rotini or shells) or rice with chunks of leftover grilled chicken or fish, whatever leftover steamed or roasted vegetables you have on hand (such as peas, broccoli, asparagus, green beans, or carrots), and some Italian salad dressing or vinaigrette.

☞ SEE ALSO MY RECIPE FOR SALMON AND ROTINI SALAD ON PAGE 202

LET'S TAKE A CLOSER LOOK

Is Microwaving Food Safe?

There's a persistent myth that microwaving destroys nutrients or alters or "denatures" food in some particularly harmful way. All cooking degrades nutrients to some extent, but microwaving foods is no more harmful than any other cooking method. In fact, the latest research indicates that microwaving is a good way to preserve the vitamin content because the food cooks quickly and with a minimum of water. However, I strongly recommend avoiding the use of plastics in the microwave—even those that are labeled "microwave safe." Use only glass or ceramic microwave-safe dishes and lids. For best results, cover cooking dishes and stir foods during cooking to ensure even heating and to avoid overcooking foods.

Cook Once, Eat Twice

Whenever you make a pot of soup, stew, or chili for dinner, pack up a couple of single-serving containers to eat for lunch later in the week. If you're not going to get to it within three or four days, freeze it in freezer-proof containers. (Don't forget to leave a little extra space at the top of the container to allow for expansion.) It's also a good idea to label freezer containers with the date and what's inside. Frozen food is good for three to four months.

Make Time for Break Time

Finally, just because you've brought your lunch with you doesn't mean you have to eat it at your desk. Step away from your work space, suspend your multitasking, and give yourself a real break. You'll enjoy your food more, improve your digestion, and return to work refreshed and ready to focus. You'll also get fewer crumbs in your keyboard.

CARRY-OUT AND CASUAL DINING

No doubt there will also be times when you'll want to grab lunch at a restaurant, deli, or carry-out place. Restaurant meals contain, on average, twice as many calories as the meals we prepare for ourselves, due to larger portion sizes and more caloric preparations. In fact, there's a direct correlation between how often you eat in restaurants and how likely you are to become overweight. The more often you eat out, the more savvy you need to be about navigating menus. Here are some tips that will help you choose wisely when eating out.

CHINESE TAKEOUT—Chinese restaurants often cater to Western tastes, emphasizing fried dishes, oversized portions, and heavy sauces. It's possible to get a healthy meal, but you need to order carefully. Avoid the fried rice, egg rolls, crispy noodles, battered and deep-fried items, and entrees with heavy sauces, such as Kung Pao, General Tso, and sweet-and-sour dishes. Instead, choose wonton or hot-and-sour soup and a spring roll, or a steamed dish with a light sauce and plain or brown rice. Most kitchens will prepare your dish with less oil and/or with extra vegetables upon request. If the portions are large (and they almost always are), split your order with a friend or pack up half for another meal.

MEXICAN—Skip the nacho chips, overstuffed burritos, and cheese-heavy quesadillas. And don't kid yourself about that taco salad: Two cups of shredded lettuce cannot redeem 1,500 calories worth of meat sauce, cheese, sour cream, and the giant deep-fried "bowl." Choose grilled chicken or vegetable fajitas, fish tacos, or tamales instead. Fresh salsa, pico de gallo, and picante sauces add flavor (and vegetables!) without a lot of calories. Portion sizes can also be a hazard at Mexican restaurants. Order your items á la carte instead of the platters that come piled high with rice and refried beans.

INDIAN—Home-cooked Indian cuisine can be quite healthful but in restaurants, the menus tend to emphasize fried foods and creamy sauces. Steer clear of the samosas, pakoras, creamed spinach, korma, and masala sauces. Instead, order tandoori or tikka dishes or make a meal out of lentil soup, roti (a whole-wheat flat bread), and raita (yogurt sauce). Although the all-you-can-eat buffet may appeal to your thrifty nature, it's a bad investment in your health—especially if you're out to get your money's worth.

SUSHI—Japanese food is among the lighter options but don't let sushi's superhealthy reputation lead you astray. Although the fresh fish and vegetables are lovely, the rice adds a surprising number of largely empty calories. You might be surprised to learn that a California roll has more calories than a fast-food hamburger. Start with miso soup or edamame (steamed soybeans) to take the edge off of your appetite and then keep it to one sushi roll or a few pieces of sashimi. Avoid tempura and sushi rolls made with fried fish, creamy sauces, or cheese. Order your sushi rolls with brown rice when you can.

DELI AND SANDWICH SHOPS—Hot, grilled sandwiches and paninis are usually extremely high in fat; avoid them. To keep from going over your calorie budget, stick to wraps or sandwiches on whole-grain bread. Choose leaner meats like turkey or roast beef and pile on the vegetables. Go easy on mayo and other creamy dressings and skip the bacon and extra cheese. Opt for coleslaw or a side salad rather than chips.

FAST FOOD AND BURGERS—Take a pass on the double-decker sandwiches, fried chicken and fish, and bacon and blue cheese toppings. A grilled chicken sandwich or veggie burger is often the best option. If you can't walk into a fast-food restaurant without ordering fries, it's best not to venture in more than once or twice a year.

ITALIAN AND PIZZA—With pasta dishes, avoid heavy, cream-based sauces like alfredo and carbonara and super-cheesy casseroles like lasagna or stuffed shells. Marinara and primavera sauces are your best choices. Say yes to the bottomless bowl of salad but no to the endless garlic bread. With pizza, steer clear of thick or filled crusts, deep-dish pies, meat-heavy toppings, and extra cheese. Look for the thin-crust, brickoven-style pizzas, topped with tomato sauce and vegetables.

Quick and Dirty Guide to Carry-out

CUISINE	CHOOSE	AVOID
Chinese	hot and sour soup wonton soup steamed spring roll chicken skewers dishes made with steamed or boiled chicken or shrimp steamed or stir-fried vegetables (request less oil)	battered or fried appetizers egg rolls General Tso's and Kung Pao chicken duck hoisin or sweet and sour sauce
Mexican	gazpacho chicken or vegetable fajitas grilled seafood dishes soft tacos tamales	chips guacamole nachos chimichangas quesadillas

CUISINE	CHOOSE	AVOID
	black beans salsa, picante, pico de gallo sauces	sopapillas crunchy tacos refried beans taco salads sour cream
Indian	tandoori roti steamed rice raita sauce lentil soup tikka	pakora samosas saag (creamed spinach) fried dishes coconut curries masala korma poori bread
Sushi	edamame miso soup sashimi seaweed salad cucumber salad	tempura or fried rolls like the spider roll, Philly roll, and spicy rolls
Deli	turkey roast beef veggie sandwiches wraps whole-wheat bread	grilled sandwiches paninis potato chips
Fast Food	grilled chicken coleslaw side salad fruit/yogurt parfait	double-decker burgers fried chicken or fish French fries onion rings fried desserts
Italian/Pizza	marinara primavera salads vegetable antipasti thin-crust pizza	carbonara alfredo garlic bread lasagna stuffed shells deep-dish pizzas meat toppings

The Chain Gang: Eating Well in Chain Restaurants

One advantage to the big national restaurant chains like Subway, Quiznos, Panera Bread, Chipotle, and Ruby Tuesday is that most of them have extensive nutritional information posted on their Web sites. Some even have tools that allow you to build your own meal before you go, adding and subtracting ingredients to see how this affects the nutritional makeup of your meal.

Though the nutrition information you see on Web sites can be helpful for giving you a general idea of the nutritional content of food, you should take it with a grain of salt. When preparing a sample dish for analysis, ingredients are precisely measured. But dishes are probably not going to be as carefully executed in the heat of battle as they were for nutrition analysis. Unless it's a highly automated fast-food restaurant where every squirt of special sauce is premeasured, you may get portions that are significantly larger, cooked in more oil or butter, and served with more salt, sauce, or salad dressing than the version that was analyzed. Nonetheless, you can use the analyses to see how the various menu items compare and zero in on the healthiest options. If you're headed to a large chain, do your research and decide what you're going to order before you go.

Working the Salad Bar

All-you-can eat buffets are popular at lunchtime but they are almost always a bad choice—especially for those who like to get their money's worth. All-you-can-eat is almost always more-than-you-should. Salad bars are the one possible exception—but even here, you can get into trouble. Here's a guide to building a healthy salad without blowing your calorie budget.

Quick and Dirty Guide to the Salad Bar

PILE IT ON	ADD SPARINGLY	JUST WALK ON BY
greens	corn	croutons
spinach	pickled beets	bacon bits
cabbage	coleslaw	chow mein noodles
tomatoes	avocado	creamy or sweet salads or relishes
cucumbers	crumbled blue cheese	creamy dressings

PILE IT ON	ADD SPARINGLY	JUST WALK ON BY
broccoli	parmesan cheese	
shredded carrots	toasted sunflower seeds	
mushrooms	slivered almonds	
onions	olives	
garbanzo beans	marinated artichokes or other	
kidney beans	vegetables	
edamame	three-bean salad	
chopped eggs	raisins	
hearts of palm	oil and vinegar dressing	
celery		
hot peppers		

HOW MUCH SHOULD YOU EAT FOR LUNCH?

Lunch should account for about one-third of your calories for the day. For most people that's somewhere between five and eight hundred calories. It's also okay to split that amount of food between a smaller lunch and a midafternoon snack—and there's much more on snacking coming up in the next chapter. You can use online nutrition information from restaurants or the Serving Size Guide at the back of the book to build the right size lunch. Here are some suggestions:

Healthy Lunches

MENU	CALORIES (APPROX.)
Tofu Salad with Nutritional Yeast sandwich (recipe on page 203) on whole-grain bread coleslaw peach	500
bowl of minestrone soup green salad with pear, blue cheese, and walnuts whole-grain roll	600
turkey, swiss, and avocado sandwich Asian-style Broccoli Salad (recipe on page 204)	700
two fish tacos with shredded cabbage, salsa, and guacamole side of black beans and rice	800

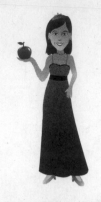

CHAPTER SIX

Snacking Well

JUST A COUPLE of generations ago, snacking between meals was considered to be an unhealthy habit. In some cultures, this is still the case. The French, for example, rarely eat between meals. They do not keep energy bars in their desk drawers. They don't sit in front of the TV with a bag of chips. And they certainly don't stroll around Le Bon Marché clutching a giant, greasy pretzel. They may be onto something. Despite the rich cuisine for which they are so famous, obesity rates in France are one-third that of what they are in the United States.

SNACKING IS OPTIONAL

Here in the United States, it's gotten to the point that we now eat pretty much constantly—in the car, at our desks, at the movies, and while we shop. I've even seen people eat during their workouts at the gym! Snacking has become so institutionalized that most "nutritious" meal plans now include three meals and at least two snacks. In fact, many people now view snacking as a nutritional necessity.

Countless diet gurus and personal trainers insist that you must eat every two to three hours to keep your metabolism revved up. However, just because you've read or heard this a few thousand times doesn't make it true. Not only will your metabolism not slow down if you go more than three hours without food, but there may actually be some benefits to going longer between meals.

LET'S TAKE A CLOSER LOOK

Metabolism Myths and Mix-ups

The popular notion that eating every few hours will keep your metabolism revved up is based on a couple of different misunderstandings about how metabolism works. The first has to do with the so-called starvation mode.

If you go too long without eating, your body adjusts its metabolism to conserve energy and burn fewer calories, just in case the food shortage continues. Going into "starvation mode" is a survival strategy. During a famine you'd need to live on your stored fat and down-regulating your metabolism is a way to make those fat stores go a bit farther. It's similar to the way your laptop adjusts its energy usage when it's running on batteries, such as by making the screen a little dimmer. When food is plentiful again, your metabolism goes back to normal, just the way your screen gets brighter when you plug your laptop back in.

If there actually were a famine, you'd be glad that your body is designed this way. But if you're trying to maintain your weight or lose a few pounds, the last thing you want is increased fuel efficiency. You want to be burning through stored fat like an Escalade burns through a tank of gas. And supposedly, if you reassure your body that there is no shortage of food by eating every few hours, it will oblige you by continuing to burn calories with reckless metabolic abandon.

The argument makes sense, except for one small thing. Your body doesn't go into starvation mode if you go three hours without food. It takes about three days of fasting or serious caloric restriction for your body to respond with any sort of metabolic adjustment.

The other misunderstanding has to do with the *thermic effect of* food. This is a term that scientists use to describe the energy that your body expends digesting your food. Think of it as a sort of transaction tax that your body charges you to convert the energy in your food into a form of energy that your cells can use. If a meal contains 300 calories worth of food energy, converting that food energy into cellular energy might use up 30 calories or so. So you'd end up with just 270 calories worth of energy when it's all over. It's a little like changing money in a foreign country. When you convert money into a different currency, you have to pay the money-changer a fee.

Some people have mistakenly interpreted this to mean that if your body is constantly in the process of digesting food, it will constantly be burning calories (due to the thermic effect of food) and that if you go too long between meals, you will be missing out on this calorie-burning opportunity. Some even go so far as to claim that you can burn more calories simply by eating more often.

This is simply a misunderstanding of how the thermic effect of food works. Just like at the money changer, the fee to exchange food energy into body energy is simply a percentage of how much you're changing. It doesn't matter whether you exchange all your money in one lump sum at the beginning of your trip or change small amounts of money three times a day. The fees will be based on how much money you convert. And the thermic effect of food is based on how much you eat, not when you eat it. Rest assured that going four—or even twelve—hours between meals will have virtually no effect on your metabolism.

What about Blood Sugar?

You'll also hear people say that eating small, frequent meals helps to keep your blood sugar levels steady. And it does: It keeps your blood sugar steadily *high*. Whoever said that your blood sugar levels were supposed to remain constant throughout the day, anyway? Blood-sugar levels naturally rise after meals, as food is digested and converted into glucose, and then fall back to baseline as the glucose is taken up by the cells and used for energy or stored for future use.

Having your blood-sugar level return to baseline is not bad for you! In fact, having your blood sugar closer to baseline for more of the day helps to protect you from developing diabetes. Now, of course, it is possible for blood sugar to get too low, which is known as hypoglycemia. A lot of people self-diagnose themselves with this condition, but very few of them actually have it. Diabetics using insulin or people with a medical condition called reactive hypogly-cemia need to be careful about letting their blood sugar get too low.

But for the vast majority of us, managing blood-sugar levels is about avoiding the peaks, not the valleys. If you experience head-aches, fatigue, and other discomfort whenever you go more than two or three hours without eating, the problem is probably not that your blood sugar has gotten too low, but that it's *been too high*. Eating a lot of sweets, sweetened beverages, white bread, and other refined carbohydrates will cause your blood sugar to go up very high, very quickly. What goes up, must come down and the higher the spike, the more uncomfortable the plunge. The easiest way to make that feeling go away is to eat again. But if you eat more of the same kinds of foods, you're simply getting back on the same roller coaster—and putting yourself on a fast track to type 2 diabetes.

To get off this roller coaster, eat foods that contain less sugar and more fiber, protein, and fat, such as whole grains, nuts, fruits, and vegetables. Your blood-sugar levels will rise more slowly and gradu-ally, making the decline far less dramatic. And you may find that you don't need to eat every three hours in order to feel well.

THE QUICK AND DIRTY SECRET

Foods that contain protein, fiber, and fat, such as whole grains, nuts, fruits, and vegetables, help keep your blood sugar from "crashing" after meals.

Benefits of Eating Less Frequently

In fact, going longer between meals can have some very beneficial effects on your blood sugar and other aspects of your health. It takes about three hours for your body to finish digesting a meal. If you eat every two or three hours, as everyone insists you should, your body will constantly be in what nutritionists call the "fed state." That simply means that you are always in the process of digesting food.

If, on the other hand, you don't eat again, you'll go into something we call the "postabsorptive state" after about three hours. Several interesting things happen in the postabsorptive state, which continues for another twelve to eighteen hours if you don't eat again. First, you begin tapping into your body's stored energy reserves to run your engine. Your hormone levels adjust to shift your body out of fat-storage mode and into fat-burning mode. Hanging out in the postabsorptive state also reduces free-radical damage and inflammation, increases the production of antiaging hormones, and promotes tissue repair. And, of course, your metabolic rate remains unchanged.

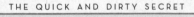

THE QUICK AND DIRTY SECRET

You don't need to worry about eating every three hours; going longer between meals is not unhealthy and can even have beneficial effects.

Feeling Hungry Is OK

The biggest problem you are likely to experience if you go a bit longer between meals is feeling hungry, and this is not as big a problem as many of us have led ourselves to believe. When you are used to always being in the fed state, you tend to panic the minute you notice that your stomach is empty. In fact, feeling hungry is not a medical emergency. Often, if you simply wait ten minutes, the feeling will go away. Sometimes simply having a cup of tea or a glass of water does the trick. Allowing your stomach to be empty for an hour or two is really not that uncomfortable if you let yourself get used to the sensation. It's also the perfect time to exercise. Exercising two or three hours after you eat will allow you to get the most out of your workout and, as a bonus, usually makes hunger pangs go away. Don't misunderstand what I'm saying here: I'm not advising you to stop eating or to starve yourself. But as long as you are eating the appropriate amount of food each day, it's okay to feel hungry between meals.

I'm not against snacking, per se—I'm an enthusiastic snacker myself. But contrary to what you may have been led to believe, snacking is definitely optional. And when you choose to snack, you want to be sure you're doing it well.

HOW TO SNACK PROPERLY

Some people find that eating five or six times a day instead of the traditional three square meals works better for them. For example, you may make better dietary choices if you don't let yourself get as hungry between meals. If that helps you maintain a healthy diet, it's a valid option. Just don't let the metabolism myth (see page 143) seduce you into thinking that eating more frequently allows you to eat more. If you're gaining weight when you don't mean to (or not losing when you're trying to), it's a sign that you need to cut back on the size of your meals or the number of your snacks (or both).

How Big Should Your Snacks Be?

The total number of calories you need to eat over the course of the day remains the same, whether you eat every five hours or every two. For most people, that's somewhere between 1,500 and 2,500 calories a day (or more if you burn a lot of calories exercising). For example, if you were to eat three meals a day with no snacking, each meal would represent roughly a third of your daily calorie budget— somewhere between 500 and 800 calories each. If you're going to eat three meals as well as a couple of snacks, you'll need to shave off a hundred or so calories from each meal and keep your snacks fairly small. If you've embraced the six-small-meals-a-day plan, then each meal should be half-sized. See the chart below for some examples of what I mean.

What's the Right-size Meal and Snack?

MEAL PLAN	SAMPLE MEAL	SAMPLE SNACK
Three Meals, No Snacks	bowl of minestrone soup green salad with pear, blue cheese, and walnuts whole-grain roll (about 600 calories)	None
Three Meals, Plus Snacks	bowl of minestrone soup green salad with blue cheese whole-grain roll (about 400 calories)	pear and walnuts (about 200 calories)
Six Small Meals	bowl of minestrone soup whole-grain roll (about 300 calories)	green salad with blue cheese, pear, and walnuts (about 300 calories)

THE QUICK AND DIRTY SECRET

The more often you eat, the smaller your meals need to be.

What Should You Snack On?

There's no shortage of snacking possibilities. You'll find munchies in every conceivable shape, size, and flavor: salty, sweet, crunchy, chewy, or all of the above. Unapologetically decadent, reduced-guilt, or earnestly virtuous, they fill several aisles of the typical grocery store, spilling out onto endcaps and lining the checkout lanes. Nor do you have to go to the grocery store to buy them. Every gas station, convenience store, shoe store, newsstand, video store, and pharmacy now doubles as a snack depot.

Not only are they cheap, convenient, and available everywhere you look, but snack foods are literally engineered to be irresistible. They're typically high in sugar, sodium, and fat—three chemicals that light up the pleasure centers of our brains and provoke mindless overeating. Once those neurotransmitters get humming, it's very hard to hear the more muffled hormonal signals that register fullness and signal you to stop eating. All too often, the bottom of the bag is the only thing that stops you. That's why I suggest that you buy (and eat) "snack foods" infrequently and in the smallest possible packages.

Instead, snack on real food—the same sort of foods that you'd eat at meals. Fresh fruits, raw vegetables, small portions of cheese, yogurt, or nuts all make convenient, portable snacks. And unlike "snack foods," real foods actually contribute to your nutritional well-being instead of subtracting from it.

SNACK ON VEGETABLES—One of the biggest challenges most people have with their diets is getting the recommended five servings of vegetables every day. Although they usually contribute only a small percentage of your daily calories, veggies are where the lion's share of the nutrients are—particularly antioxidants and other cancer-fighting, antiaging, and generally good-for-you compounds.

Snacks offer the perfect opportunity to wedge another serving or two of vegetables into your day. Rather than reaching for pretzels or chips, crunch on raw veggies instead. Baby carrots, grape tomatoes, radishes, snow peas, and sugar snap peas are convenient and portable, and don't require any cutting or peeling. Raw cauliflower florets, red peppers strips, celery sticks, cucumber rounds, or zucchini spears take just a few minutes more to prepare. Because they are so low in calories, you can eat as many raw vegetables as you like. But to make your snack go a bit farther, add a moderate amount (a third of a cup) of a healthy dip like hummus, guacamole, or tapenade.

☛ SEE MY RECIPE FOR TOMATILLO GUACAMOLE ON PAGE 207

Get More Nutrition from Vegetables

Most vegetables are fat-free but many of the most valuable nutrients in vegetables are fat-soluble vitamins. These include vitamin A, which protects your eyesight; vitamin K, which builds healthy bones and keeps your heart healthy; as well as beta carotene, lycopene, and all the carotenoids, which fight free radicals and ward off cancer.

In order to be absorbed into your cells, where they can do you some good, these nutrients need to hitch a ride on a fat molecule. Eating your spinach sauteed in a bit of olive oil and garlic or dipping your carrot sticks in peanut butter is actually much better for you than eating them plain. A study published in the *Journal of Nutrition* reported that when researchers added avocado to a salad, the subjects absorbed up to fifteen times more fat-soluble nutrients than those who ate the plain salad.

SNACK ON FRUIT—Fresh fruit is also a good source of fiber, antioxidants, vitamins, and minerals. But unlike vegetables, fruit is fairly high in sugar, so you don't want to overdo it. Two cups of fruit a day is a good rule of thumb. A cup is about the size of your fist. An average-size apple, orange, or banana would count as a cup. For apricots or plums, two would count as a cup. If you're the type that tends to crave sweet snacks, I suggest you use your fruit allowance to satisfy that urge. And if you're not a big fan of fruit, you can eat a couple of extra servings of vegetables instead; both food groups supply the same type of nutrients.

You'll get the most nutritional value from fresh, whole fruit—ideally whatever is local and in season. Dried fruit such as apricots, figs, and raisins are a convenient alternative. Just bear in mind that the portion sizes for dried fruit are a lot smaller. A quarter cup of raisins or a third of a cup of dried apricots, prunes, or apple slices is equal to one cup of fresh fruit. Fruit juice is the least nutritious option. In fact, when it comes to fruit juice, less really is more. Despite its seemingly wholesome origins, most fruit juice is high in sugar and low in nutrients and fiber. The new fruit-and-vegetable juice blends are really no better. Research shows that people who drink more fruit *juice* have a higher risk of developing type 2 diabetes. Yet, eating more *whole* fruit decreases that risk.

THE QUICK AND DIRTY SECRET

If you prefer vegetables, it's fine to substitute them for fruit. Both food groups contain the same nutrients.

LET'S TAKE A CLOSER LOOK

Should Fruit Always Be Eaten by Itself?

Contrary to what you may have heard, there is no reason that you need to eat fruit separate from all other kinds of food. The notion that fruit should always be eaten by itself is a variation on the food combining myth I talked about on page 133. Like so many nutrition myths, this one has a kernel of truth. It's true that fruit passes through your stomach and into the small intestine more slowly if you eat with other foods than it does when you eat it all by itself. But it's not true that this causes the fruit to ferment in your stomach. Your stomach is far too acidic for any fermentation to occur. On the contrary, pairing fruit with a small serving (an ounce or so) of nuts or cheese is an excellent idea. Foods that contain protein and/or healthy fats help to slow down the absorption of sugar from fruit. Instead of a short-lived burst of energy that leaves you hungry an hour later, you'll get a few hours of appetite control and steady energy. See page 153 for some classic combinations.

Pair fruit with a small serving of nuts or cheese to avoid a sharp rise (and fall) in blood sugar.

SNACK ON CHEESE—A one-ounce serving of cheese contains roughly the same amount of fat, calories, protein, and calcium as an eight-ounce serving of whole milk. Low-fat cheeses are comparable to low-fat milk. Just keep in mind that a serving of cheese is a whole lot smaller than a serving of milk, because most of the fluid has been drained off or pressed out of it. Although it provides healthy nutrients like protein and calcium, because it is high in fat, cheese can also be a concentrated source of calories. If you're trying to gain weight, cheese can be a good way to get extra calories into your diet. If you're not, keep an eye on your portion sizes.

What's a Serving of Cheese?

1 ounce of hard cheese = size of your thumb or a compact disc (without case)

1 ounce of soft cheese = size of a ping-pong ball

1 ounce of crumbled or shredded cheese = size of a large egg

1 ounce of grated cheese = size of a tangerine or clementine

1 ounce of melted cheese = enough to fill a shot glass

SNACK ON NUTS—Nuts pack a whole lot of nutrition into a small package—which makes them ideal for on-the-go snacking. They're rich in antioxidants, fiber, and heart-healthy fats. They also contain nutrients called plant sterols, which help to lower LDL (or "bad") cholesterol. However, nuts are also notoriously calorie-packed. If you're not paying attention, you can easily inhale a meal's worth of calories in a couple of minutes without even realizing it. Although nuts have a lot going for them nutritionally, you still need to pay attention to the portion size (unless you're *trying* to gain weight). A serving of nuts (approximately 100 calories) is one ounce. For larger nuts like almonds or walnuts, an ounce is about twenty nuts. For smaller nuts, like peanuts or pistachios, an ounce is around thirty nuts. Two table-spoons of nut butter counts as a serving. Pair nuts with fresh or dried fruit or enjoy them all by themselves.

THE QUICK AND DIRTY SECRET

Nuts are a healthy snack but also a concentrated source of calo-ries. Enjoy them in small portions—especially if weight control is a concern.

Healthy 200-Calorie(ish) Snacks

Slice ½ apple and spread with 2 tablespoons peanut butter (or other nut butter)

Combine 4–6 dried apricots (or figs) with 20 roasted cashews (or almonds)

Classic GORP: 2 tablespoons raisins and 2 tablespoons dry-roasted peanuts

Dip raw vegetables in ⅓ cup hummus or Tomatillo Guacamole (recipe on page 207)

Spread cucumber slices with ¼ cup goat cheese spread (recipe for Goat Cheese Spread with Fig and Black Pepper on page 208)

Toss ½ cup grapefruit sections with ½ cup cubed avocado

Top ½ cup cottage cheese with ¾ cup fresh pineapple or melon balls

Should You Eat Energy Bars?

Although I think it's always preferable to snack on real food, there are all kinds of energy and meal replacement bars designed to offer a convenient solution to your on-the-go nutrition needs. They don't need refrigeration, preparation, or even utensils. In a pinch, they will keep you going. But it's important to match the bar to the situation. For example, if it's three P.M. and you're sitting at your desk feeling a little groggy, it might seem like an energy bar would be the perfect solution. But unless your job involves heavy physical work, that's not really the kind of energy you're looking for. More likely, you could use a break, a walk, a stretch, some fresh air, a cup of tea or maybe even a power nap. Any of these will be more energizing than a concentrated dose of carbohydrates.

Here's a guide to the different types of bars and when to choose them:

SPORT NUTRITION—Energy or sport bars like Clif Bars and Power-Bars are designed for athletes who need a convenient way to carry a concentrated source of calories (or *food energy*) on long workouts. They are usually high in simple carbohydrates (otherwise known as sugar) because that's the sort of fuel that can be most efficiently converted into muscle energy during exercise. They may contain some protein but they usually don't contain a whole lot of fat because it takes the body a long time to convert fat to energy. It may seem as if a product designed for athletes would be a particularly healthy choice, but unless you're involved in lengthy vigorous exercise, a concentrated dose of simple carbohydrates is the last thing you want. (See also "Nutrition and Exercise," on page 189.)

THE QUICK AND DIRTY SECRET

High-carbohydrate sports bars only make sense when you're engaged in heavy-duty exercise.

MEAL REPLACEMENT—If you're using a bar to stand in for a meal or snack, skip the sport and granola bars, which tend to be mostly carbohydrates. Instead, look for bars with a balance of protein, carbohydrates, and fats, and a healthy dose of fiber. Because fat and protein take longer to digest, including some in your meal keeps you from getting hungry again so quickly. Fiber helps slow down the absorption of sugars and carbohydrates, which helps keeps your blood sugar and energy steadier. The Nutrition Facts label can help you gauge how balanced it is. A bar that provides 25 percent of the Daily Value for carbohydrate but only 3 percent of the Daily Value for fat or protein won't make a terribly well-balanced meal.

Although you can find bars that are higher in protein and fat, it's hard to find bars that aren't also very high in sugar. Ever notice that they don't make meal replacement bars in flavors like salmon and brown rice or broccoli and tofu? Instead, your "meal" choices are strawberry shortcake, peanut butter brownie, or chocolate caramel pretzel. Any protein or fiber the bar provides is usually all held together with the nutritional equivalent of marshmallow fluff. Wholesome-sounding ingredients like brown rice syrup, organic evaporated cane juice, grape or apple juice concentrates, and barley malt syrup are all just forms of sugar. In fact, most of these bars—even the organic, whole-grain ones—have as much sugar as the average candy bar.

THE QUICK AND DIRTY SECRET

Meal-replacement bars should be the option of last resort; they make a poor substitute for a healthy meal.

LOW-CARB BARS—You'll also find low-carb bars made with artificial sweeteners and a variety of gums, resins, and other high-tech ingredients. They contain mostly protein, fiber, and fat. (This makes them almost useless as fuel for exercise, by the way.) They can be used as a low-carb meal replacement, but these highly processed bars usually bear about as much resemblance to actual food as a paper towel resembles a tree.

WHOLE FOOD BARS—Finally, there are also some bars out there that are made almost entirely with whole foods like dried fruits and nuts. Then again, wouldn't it be just as convenient (and a whole lot cheaper) to keep some dried fruit and nuts around? Or, if you've got some time, why not make your own whole-food snack bars?

☞ SEE MY RECIPE FOR BEST FRUIT AND NUT BARS ON PAGE 206

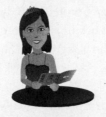

CHAPTER SEVEN

Dinner Done Right

AH, THOSE THREE dreaded words: "What's for dinner?" But there's no need to panic or despair. Thanks to your savvy shopping (see Part One), you've got everything you need to throw together a fabulous, healthy meal. And if you've been with me so far through Part Two, you're ahead of the game at this point. You don't have to figure out a way to fit all five servings of vegetables into the last meal of the day and you haven't already blown your calorie budget for the week.

It needn't take more than thirty minutes to get a real meal together. But at the end of the day, when you're hungry and tired, it's easy for good intentions to falter. Before you know it, you're halfway through a bag of potato chips and dialing for pizza. "I'll make a salad to go with the pizza," you promise yourself. But somehow the salad never happens. Believe me, I know how it goes. Instead of tearing into the chips, buy yourself some time with a snack that will take the edge off your hunger without scuttling the nutritional integrity of the whole evening. A small dish of olives, some carrots and hummus, or a glass of spicy tomato juice set the tone for a healthy dinner.

WHAT TO EAT FOR DINNER

Nutritionally speaking, dinner isn't much different from lunch. You want at least one serving of protein—and maybe more if you want take advantage of the fat-burning, appetite-regulating, and muscle-building effects of protein I mentioned in chapter 5. Your dinner protein can be meat, fish, poultry, or eggs. But don't overlook vegetarian options like tofu, lentils, or beans. Aside from the potential health benefits, vegetarian protein is usually cheaper as well as easier on the environment. Even without becoming a full-time vegetarian, you can save money on your grocery bill and reduce your carbon footprint by eating meatless more often. In addition to protein, dinner should include a serving or two of vegetables and, perhaps, some sort of grain or starch. Check the Serving Size Guide on page 232 for a guide to portion sizes.

KITCHEN TIP

Dried Bean Time Saver

I like to use dried rather than canned beans in soups and chili because they are lower in sodium and have a better flavor and texture (they're also cheaper!). But soaking and precooking dried beans requires a certain amount of planning ahead. Fortunately, cooked beans freeze really well. Next time you're soaking and boiling dried beans, prepare double what your recipe calls for and freeze what you don't use. The next time you need precooked (or canned) beans, whip them out of the freezer and you're ready to go.

☛ SEE RECIPE FOR LOUISIANA RED BEANS AND RICE ON PAGE 219

Is a Vegetarian Diet Healthier?

Many studies have shown that vegetarians are less likely to be overweight; have lower rates of cancer, heart disease, and many other diseases; and tend to live longer. But studies like this look backward in time. They tell you how yesterday's vegetarians fared compared with yesterday's carnivores. That doesn't necessarily tell you how today's vegetarians will fare in the future—especially because vegetarianism has become a completely different game than it was twenty or thirty years ago.

The percentage of true vegetarians hasn't changed that much over the last three decades. But the percentage of people who choose vegetarian options some of the time has skyrocketed. And, because it exists to satisfy your every desire, commerce has risen to the challenge. Twenty years ago, if you wanted rice milk or vegan mayonnaise, you had to shop in a health food coop. Today, you can walk into any gas station convenience store and find soy creamer for your coffee.

But the more mainstream vegetarianism gets, the less healthy it seems to become. The typical vegan or vegetarian diet used to include more fruits, vegetables, whole grains, beans, and legumes, and less sugar, salt, and saturated fat than the typical omnivore's fare. Today's vegan, however, can easily get through the entire day without coming close to a fresh vegetable. You can fill your cart with vegan frozen pizzas, burritos, and waffles; fake bacon, sausage, and hot dogs; cookies, cakes, and donuts; chips, dips, crackers, and fake cheese; and vegan breakfast cereals that make Cap'n Crunch look virtuous—without venturing beyond a mainstream grocery store.

People sometimes think that if they're eating only or mostly vegetarian or vegan products, their diet is automatically going to be healthier. Obviously, however, a diet of vegan junk food isn't going to be any better for you than a diet of regular junk food.

Whether you're vegan, vegetarian, or a meat-eater, your diet will only be as healthy as you make it. And the rules are basically the same for everyone.

- Eat a balanced and varied diet that meets your nutritional needs. For vegetarians, it's particularly important to ensure that you're getting enough iron, vitamin B12, and zinc. Contrary to popular belief, however, vegetarians generally don't need to worry about getting enough protein or combining certain foods to produce "complete" proteins.

- Eat plenty of fresh vegetables.
- Don't eat too much. No matter what kind of foods you do or don't eat, it's important to maintain a healthy weight.
- Limit your consumption of processed foods, which tend to be high in sugar and salt.

HOW TO COOK MEAT

I'm a big fan of grilling at supper time. It's quick, easy, delicious, and (woo-hoo!) creates a lot fewer dishes to wash. You don't have to use any added fat to get great flavor and a good bit of the fat actually drips away during the grilling process. There is, however, a snag. Grilling meat over gas flames or charcoal can promote the formation of harmful chemicals called heterocyclic amines (HCAs) and polycyclic aromatic hydrocarbons (PAHs). The former are caused when amino acids in meat (including poultry and fish) are subjected to high temperatures; the latter form when fat from the meat drips down onto hot surfaces and flares up. HCAs and PAHs are both known carcinogens. Fortunately, you can dramatically reduce the formation of HCAs and PAHs by making a few simple (and in some cases, tasty) adjustments to your grilling technique. See How to Grill Meat Safely on the following page.

Because they both involve very high temperatures, broiling and frying are also likely to produce HCAs in meat. You can minimize this somewhat by broiling meat under (not over) the heat source and making sure that any drippings can drain into a broiler pan where they are less likely to flame up. Fried foods are not only high in HCAs but high in unhealthy trans fats and are best avoided. Baking, stewing, poaching, and braising are all healthy ways to cook meat because the meat cooks at lower temperatures. See page 233 for a guide to cooking methods.

Worry-free Grilling

Grilling vegetables, tofu, or veggie burgers does not create HCAs or PAHs. And indoor grills, such as the popular George Foreman grills, do not present the same dangers as outdoor grilling because the temperatures tend to be lower and there is no flame to cause flare-ups or smoke.

How to Grill Meat Safely

Minimize time on the grill. For foods that take longer to cook (such as whole chicken breasts) or are higher in fat (such as pork or lamb chops), partially precooking them in the microwave and finishing them on the grill can vastly reduce the formation of harmful compounds.

Don't let fat drip onto hot surfaces. If you get a flare-up, immediately move the meat to a cooler area of the grill or off the grill entirely until the flames are out. Indirect cooking methods, such as piling charcoals to one side of the grill and cooking on the other side or turning the gas burner directly under the meat down or off can also help prevent flare-ups.

Don't let meats get heavily charred or blackened. Use a lower flame or smaller pile of charcoal to keep the grill from getting too hot.

Use marinades and spice rubs. Marinating meat in a marinade containing some form of acid (wine, vinegar, citrus, Worcestershire sauce, etc.) for thirty minutes before grilling can block over 90 percent of HCA formation. To avoid flare-ups, use marinades that are low in oil, and to keep foods from getting overly blackened, avoid sauces that are high in sugar. Adding herbs and spices like rosemary, oregano, ginger, garlic, or cloves to your marinade or to the meat itself also powerfully blocks the formation of HCAs and other harmful chemicals.

☛ SEE RECIPE FOR MOROCCAN SLIDERS, PAGE 217

☛ YOU'LL FIND SOME OF MY FAVORITE MAIN DISH RECIPES, IN THE RECIPE SECTION, WHICH STARTS ON PAGE 197

HOW TO COOK VEGETABLES

Whenever you cook foods, some nutrients—especially water soluble vitamins and antioxidants—are destroyed by heat. Other nutrients, including minerals, may leach out into cooking water. Keep in mind, however, that nutrients are also lost when foods are washed, frozen, cut up, blended, or dehydrated—or even just stored. According to the USDA, freshly harvested vegetables can lose up to half their original nutritional value simply by sitting on your counter for two days—or in your refrigerator for two weeks.

How Cooking Methods Affect Nutrients

Some nutrients are more affected by cooking than others. Calcium is pretty sturdy while vitamin C, folate, and potassium are quite fragile. It also depends on what kind of cooking you're doing. As a general rule, minerals can take the heat. In fact, dry heat, such as baking or roasting, hardly affects mineral content at all. Vitamins, on the other hand, seem to do slightly better with moist cooking methods, such blanching—mostly because the cooking times are shorter. Because most vegetables contain both vitamins and minerals, you'll usually have to settle for some sort of trade-off.

I think it's worth doing what you can to minimize nutrient losses. But unless you can arrange to eat every meal in the field in which it was grown, some nutrients will always be lost. This is one of those things you can stop worrying about. Even when vegetables have lost some of their nutritional value, there is still plenty of nutrition left in them. Here are tips for keeping more of the nutrients in your vegetables. See also the Guide to Cooking Methods on page 233.

MINIMIZE COOKING TIMES AND CONTACT WITH WATER—Steaming vegetables in a rack placed above boiling water keeps the vegetables out of the water, so fewer nutrients leach into the liquid. On the other hand, steaming vegetables can take up to twice as long as boiling them and the extra time can lead to additional losses of heat-sensitive nutrients. Adding vegetables to boiling water and cooking just until tender is just as good a way to preserve nutrient content. Microwaving vegetables may offer the best of both worlds because it minimizes cooking times *and* contact with water. In fact, studies show that microwaving preserves more nutrients in vegetables than other cooking methods. See also "Is Microwaving Food Safe?" on page 135.

USE THE COOKING LIQUID—When you cook foods in water or other liquids, both vitamins and minerals can leach out into the cooking liquid. If you discard the liquid, those nutrients end up going down the drain. If you can figure out a way to include the cooking liquid in the meal instead, you'll salvage a lot of that nutrition. For example, when you make vegetable soup, a lot of the nutrients from your vegetables may end up in the broth. But that's okay, because you're going to eat the broth, too. When you boil or steam vegetables, save the vitamin-rich cooking water and use it to make rice or couscous, thereby recapturing some of those nutrients.

☛ SEE THE RECIPES FOR SILKEN ASPARAGUS SOUP ON PAGE 209
AND SWEET POTATO AND CAULIFLOWER CURRY ON PAGE 210

DON'T OVERCOOK YOUR VEGETABLES—No matter how you're preparing them, overcooking vegetables increases nutrient losses. When making a soup or stew, add vegetables that require longer cooking times, such as carrots, early on and those that cook quickly, such as zucchini, at the end. Likewise, when cooking broccoli, separate the florets from the stems and add them to the boiling water (or steamer basket) a few minutes after you start cooking the stems. That way, they'll all be done at the same time and you'll keep more of the vitamins in your veggies.

☛ SEE THE RECIPE FOR ASIAN-STYLE BROCCOLI SALAD
ON PAGE 204

EAT SOME RAW—Because nutrients are inevitably lost in cooking, at least some of the fruits and vegetables you eat each day should ideally be eaten raw.

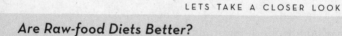

LETS TAKE A CLOSER LOOK

Are Raw-food Diets Better?

Some people advocate raw food diets, made up mostly or entirely of foods that are not cooked. Proponents of this diet argue that cooking foods destroys nutrients. They also claim that raw foods contain enzymes which help us digest our food and enhance nutrient absorption. While I think that you can get a lot of nutritional benefit from eating raw fruits and vegetables, I don't think you need to stop cooking all of your food in order to have a healthy diet.

For one thing, raw foods are not *necessarily* more nutritious. Foods lose nutrients over time, even if they are never cooked. In fact, frozen vegetables that are processed immediately after harvest can be more nutritious than raw vegetables that have been in transit or sitting in your fridge for a couple of weeks. Second, just because the foods eaten in a raw food diet aren't *cooked*, that doesn't mean they're not *processed*. On the contrary, foods may be dried, rolled, juiced, blended, frozen, soaked, sprouted, fermented, or ground—all of which may involve nutrient losses.

Finally, there's little evidence to indicate that the enzymes in raw foods are beneficial—probably because they are unlikely to survive the acidic environment of the stomach. The enzymes in raw vegetables no doubt served very important functions when those plants were living. But whether or not they've been deactivated by heat or by your stomach acid, the enzymes in your food function primarily as a source of amino acids (or protein) that your body can use to produce its own enzymes, as needed.

☛ YOU'LL FIND MORE OF MY FAVORITE WAYS TO PREPARE VEGETABLES IN THE RECIPE SECTION, WHICH STARTS ON PAGE 197

GRAINS AND OTHER STARCHES

Carbohydrate foods like bread, grains, and pasta are widely feared and mistrusted these days and many would argue that they have no place on your dinner plate. Although I agree that you should choose your carbohydrates wisely and avoid eating them in excessive quantities, I don't agree that you need to eliminate all grains or starches from your diet in order to be healthy.

The Institute of Medicine recommends that you get between 45 and 65 percent of your calories from carbohydrates, and that includes the carbohydrates you get from fruits, vegetables, and dairy products. If you recall from chapter 5, their recommended range for protein is 10 to 35 percent of your calories—and there's a relationship between these two. As the percentage of protein in your diet goes up, the percentage of carbohydrate goes down, and vice versa.

Here's what this means for you: If you're aiming for the higher end of the recommended range for protein intake (see "How Much Protein Should You Eat?" page 131), you'll want to aim for the lower end of the carbohydrate range. For the average-sized person, the lower end of the range translates to about four to six servings of grains or grain-based foods per day. If your protein intake is at the lower end of the range—for example, if you're a vegetarian—then your carbohydrate intake would be at the higher end of the range, or six to nine servings per day. And to remind you of a point I made in chapter 2, the more servings of grains you eat, the more important it is that most of them be whole grains.

What's a Serving of Grains?

1 piece of bread
½ cup cooked grains
½ cup cooked pasta
1 ounce dry pasta
¼ cup uncooked grains

Cooking Whole Grains

If you want to include a starch on the dinner plate, cooked whole grains like brown rice, quinoa, and wild rice are the most nutritious options. (See chapter 2 for a guide to grains.) As for preparing them, two basic cooking techniques are really all you need.

STEAMED GRAINS—Steamed grains are mildly flavored and make a good complement to dishes with a lot of flavor or sauce, such as Louisiana Red Beans and Rice, page 219, or Sweet Potato and Cauliflower Curry, page 210. Steamed grains can also be used in cold salads, such as Quinoa Salad with Pecans and Cranberries, page 214.

The basic technique for steaming grains is to measure grains and water into a saucepan with a tightly fitted lid. Some grains (such as basmati rice and quinoa) are also rinsed in cold water before cooking.

To begin, add a pinch of salt and/or a pat of butter or glug of olive oil, if desired. Then bring the water to a boil and then cover the pan tightly and turn the heat to low. Steam until all the water has been absorbed. The proportions of water to grain and the cooking time vary from grain to grain so consult the package for guidance.

THE PILAF METHOD—The pilaf method is a more flavorful preparation that makes a good accompaniment to simple grilled or roasted meat or vegetables, such as the Roasted Cauliflower on page 211 or the Moroccan Sliders on page 217.

The basic technique for pilaf is to sauté chopped vegetables (such as onions, garlic, carrots, celery, green pepper, etc.) in oil until tender. Add the dry grains and toast them briefly with the vegetables. Then add water or stock (see package for the correct proportions) and salt, if desired. Lower heat, cover tightly, and cook until water is absorbed.

Rethinking Pasta

For some reason, when it comes to pasta, we seem to suffer from some pretty crazy portion distortion. A one-cup portion of rice looks perfectly appropriate to us—even generous. But put one cup of pasta onto a dinner plate and it doesn't look right at all. Thanks to advertising and the oversized portions in restaurants, we're used to seeing portions of pasta four or five times that size. Personally, I'm a big fan of pasta and I always keep it on hand. It's inexpensive, it's fast to cook, and you can serve it a million different ways. But I have had to train myself to recalibrate the portion sizes. Instead of thinking of pasta as the main course, think of it as an accompaniment to whatever vegetables or protein you're serving with it.

☞ SEE MY RECIPE FOR PENNE WITH SAUTÉED CHARD ON PAGE 215

Pasta and Your Blood Sugar

Carbohydrate-rich foods like pasta have a high glycemic load, which means they can cause a quick rise in blood sugar. Overcooked pasta sends blood sugar higher than pasta cooked al dente. To lower its glycemic impact, cook your pasta just until tender, keep portion sizes moderate, and add some protein to the meal.

You can also make smaller portions go further by adding vegetables to the pasta itself. Try coarsely chopping some kale and adding it to the water with rotini pasta. The two take about the same length of time to cook. When both are tender, drain and top with sauce as usual. Or, combine equal parts cooked linguine and shredded spaghetti squash and you can have twice as much for virtually the same amount of carbs.

KITCHEN TIP

How to Cook Spaghetti Squash

Spaghetti squash is a variety of winter squash, related to butternut and acorn squash. Baked until tender and shredded with a fork, it turns into spaghetti-like strands. To prepare, cut spaghetti squash in half, lengthwise, and scoop out seeds and fibers. Place squash halves skin side up on a foil-covered baking sheet and place in oven at 350 degrees for forty minutes or until tender. (To test for doneness, flip the squash over and poke fork into flesh. When the squash yields easily, it is done.) Cool just until squash can be handled and then pull a fork through the squash lengthwise, shredding the squash into a bowl. Keep shredding until all the squash is removed from the shell. Discard the shells and top the squash as you would regular spaghetti.

Skip the Carbs and Get a Bonus Serving of Vegetables

Most of us have been trained to think of dinner as having three essential components: a protein, a vegetable, and a starch—such as rice, potatoes, or pasta. If you find it difficult to get five servings of vegetables every day or you're looking for a place to trim some calories, consider skipping the starch at dinner and making two vegetables instead. Instead of making chicken breasts with broccoli and rice, make chicken breasts with broccoli and baked acorn squash. It doesn't take any more time and you still have plenty of variety on your plate. Plus, you've gotten a bonus serving of vegetables. This works when you're eating out, as well. Simply ask the server if they can substitute a second vegetable for the starch. Usually, this is no problem.

HOW MUCH SHOULD YOU EAT FOR DINNER?

Dinner should take up about a third of your calories for the day. For most people that's somewhere between 500 and 800 calories. See the Serving Size Guide at the back of the book for a rough guide to portion sizes and approximate calorie counts. Below I've given some examples of healthy menus at various calorie levels.

Healthy Dinners	
MENU	CALORIES (APPROX.)
Louisiana Red Beans and Rice (recipe on page 219) garden salad with oil and vinegar dressing	500
Crunchy Sesame Flax Chicken (recipe on page 216) watermelon coleslaw baked acorn squash	600
grilled fish Braised Fennel (recipe on page 212) roasted sweet potato glass of wine	700
grilled steak Penne with Sautéed Chard (recipe on page 215) tomato salad square of dark chocolate	800

EATING DINNER OUT

Sometimes the answer to the question, "What's for Dinner?" is "Reservations!" If you're someone who eats out frequently, you should be aware that dining out is a major risk factor for weight gain. Restaurant food tends to be richer and more caloric (there's a reason it tastes so good!) and the portions are usually much larger than most people should be eating. Of course, it's possible to eat out and still have a healthy diet—but it generally doesn't happen by accident.

Restaurant Ready

One important skill is the ability to decode menu descriptions and spot the healthier dishes. The words "creamy," "crispy," and "smothered," for example, are all code for "loaded with fat." I'd also be on guard against items described as "rich," "thick," or anything topped with several kinds of cheese. Instead of dishes that get their flavor from heavy sauces, look for the simpler preparations. Words like "steamed," "seared," "poached," or "grilled" signal a lighter, leaner style of cooking.

Decoding the Menu

WORDS TO WATCH FOR	WHAT IT REALLY MEANS
all you can eat	more than you should eat
au gratin	topped with cheese, butter, bread crumbs
battered	fried
breaded	usually fried
buttery	high in fat (may or may not involve butter)
cheesy	high in fat
country-style	battered, fried, creamed, with gravy
crispy	fried
creamed/creamy	swimming in butter, milk, or cream
crusted	breaded; often fried
loaded	overloaded
smothered	smothered in calories
stuffed	overstuffed

You'll have an easier time finding healthy menu options if you pick your restaurant with that in mind. As much as I love Indian food, most Indian restaurant meals are very high in fat and calories. Sushi restaurants, however, are a great place to get a light, nutritious meal. Pub grub is usually heavy on fried foods, whereas a grill may have more healthy choices. Diners tend to specialize in things covered with cheese, gravy, or syrup; a bistro usually has entrée salads and other lighter options. Or, take advantage of the "small plate" trend by seeking out Spanish or Middle Eastern restaurants that serve tapas or mezze. Instead of ordering an entrée, you make a meal out of small "tasting" portions of three or four different dishes.

In addition, here are a couple of ordering strategies that can help you get a healthier meal without feeling like you're left nibbling nothing but garnishes:

ORDER A FIRST COURSE—You're a lot more likely to overorder (and overeat) when you're very hungry. Instead, order a salad or soup but delay ordering your entree until after you've eaten the first course.

ASK THEM TO GO LIGHTLY—Request that salads and other dishes be lightly dressed or sauced. Sauces and dressings are where all the calories hang out and most kitchens apply them with a heavy hand. Asking for things to be lightly sauced or dressed usually results in a lower-calorie plate.

INQUIRE ABOUT HALF PORTIONS—Except for nouvelle cuisine restaurants where everything is the size of an ice cube, most restaurant portions are two or three times what any normal person should be eating at a meal. Even if they are not listed on the menu, many kitchens will serve half portions upon request.

ASK FOR THE VEGGIE OF THE DAY—Most restaurants will have one or two fresh vegetables that they are serving on any given day, although they may not be listed on the menu. These can often be requested in place of potato or French fries.

WORK THE SMALL PLATES—You can turn any restaurant into a small-plate restaurant by ordering two or three appetizers as your meal.

LATE-NIGHT SNACKING

There's a popular piece of nutrition lore that says that eating before bed leads to weight gain. The idea is that calories are more readily turned to fat if you lie down after eating them. Accordingly, you're advised to stop eating early in the evening so that you have a chance to "burn off" those calories before you go to bed. Although this seems logical, there is no truth to it. Foods have the same number of calories whether you're vertical or horizontal while you're digesting them. Research on this issue confirms that what matters most is how many calories you eat over the course of the day, not when you eat them.

However, there are several good reasons to limit snacking after dinner. If you suffer from heartburn or reflux, it's best not to lie down for at least two hours after eating. Many people also find that adopting a "no eating after 8 P.M." rule helps them manage their weight. But there is no metabolic magic involved. Snacking in the evening is usually recreational eating—extra calories that we pile on after the day's nutritional needs have been met. Also, a lot of people find that their self-control is lower in the evening and they end up eating more than they mean to or indulging in foods that they wouldn't choose by the bright light of day. It's the extra calories that lead to weight gain, not the time of day that they're eaten.

If you like a snack in the evening, you'll need to budget your intake throughout the day so that you've got some calories left over for it. For example, you could choose to skip the rice or potato at dinner

and, instead, make a batch of popcorn to have as an evening snack
(see my instructions on page 97).

THE QUICK AND DIRTY SECRET

Calories that you eat in the evening aren't any more likely to make
you gain weight than calories eaten any other time of the day.

And with that, we've come to the end of the nutritional day! In the
next chapter, I cover a few nonessentials that may still deserve a
place in your healthy diet.

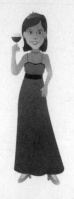

CHAPTER EIGHT

Drinks and Desserts

ALCOHOLIC BEVERAGES

Whenever my friend orders a drink or a glass of wine, he always jokes that it's "strictly for medicinal purposes" or "doctor's orders." After all, moderate alcohol consumption appears to have a number of well-publicized health benefits. On average, people who drink moderately live a little longer and are a little healthier than those who don't drink at all. Why? Mostly because moderate alcohol consumption is good for your heart. It reduces your risk of heart disease and stroke—presumably by thinning the blood and reducing inflammation. Although the cardiovascular benefits account for most of the impact on longevity, a bit of alcohol also seems to reduce the risk of many other diseases.

But—and this is a big but— this modest benefit disappears pretty quickly as alcohol consumption goes up. When you chart the relationship between alcohol consumption and mortality rates, you'll see why it's often described as a J-shaped curve. The mortality rates dip slightly as alcohol consumption increases from zero to one or two drinks a day, then rises sharply with every drink after that. If you find it difficult to drink moderately, you're really better off not

drinking at all. And if you don't drink, there's no reason to start tip-
pling just for the health benefits.

The damage caused by drinking excessively far outweighs the
benefits of drinking moderately.

How Much Alcohol Is Healthy?

The amount of alcohol that's considered healthy is one drink per day
if you're a woman and two a day if you're a man. Above that amount,
the risks outweigh the benefits. Why do men get to drink more?
Well, men are bigger on average, but it's not just about body size.
Women also metabolize alcohol differently and can tolerate less.

A drink may also be less than you think. One "drink" is defined
as 12 ounces of beer, 5 ounces of wine, or an ounce and a half of
liquor—but the typical drink served in a bar or restaurant may contain
a lot more than that. A martini can easily contain three or four drinks'
worth of alcohol and draft beers are frequently 16 to 20 ounces.

What Kind of Drink Is Healthiest?

Red wine may offer a little extra health boost in the form of polyphenols that are found in the skins of the grapes. (You can get these same
compounds in nonalcoholic grape juice, by the way.) But in terms of
overall health and longevity, beer, wine, and spirits all have about
the same benefits.

All alcoholic drinks can be a significant source of calories. Beer
ranges from 80 calories per bottle for the light and low-calorie beer,
to over 200 calories for darker, heavier, beers. Wine ranges from 120
to 160 calories per glass. Most liquors average about 120 to 150 calories a shot—and if a drink involves several shots of liquor, multiply
accordingly. Mixers and other ingredients can add several hundred
additional calories per drink—usually in the form of sugar.

Best / Worst Drink Choices

Additional health benefits: red wine, Bloody Mary
Lower in calories: dry wine, light beer, champagne, highballs made
   with soda or seltzer, classic martini (not oversized)
Lower in alcohol: mimosa, wine spritzer
High in calories, sugar, and/or alcohol: Frozen margaritas and
   daiquiris, piña coladas, kahlua and cream, white Russian, Long Island
   iced tea, chocolate and other "dessert" martinis, egg nog

THE QUICK AND DIRTY SECRET

To avoid drinking too many calories, choose lighter beers, drier
wines, and avoid frozen, fruity, creamy, and oversized drinks.

Does Cooking Burn Off Alcohol?

It's a common misconception that when you add wine or other liquor to a recipe, all of the alcohol cooks off. Although some does
evaporate, up to 85 percent of the alcohol can remain in the finished
dish! Flaming or flambéing is one of the least effective ways of removing alcohol, leaving up to 75 percent of the alcohol intact. Sim-
mering is more effective — but it takes about three hours to cook off
all of the alcohol. If an alcohol-free result is important, substitute
non-alcoholic wine, which provides much of the same flavor without any alcohol.

SWEET STUFF

Throughout this book, I've talked about the importance of limiting your intake of refined sugar and foods and beverages that contained added sugars. Although you may not immediately see or
feel the effects, a diet high in sugar accelerates the aging process—

both inside and out—and puts you on the short list for obesity, heart disease, diabetes, and cancer. That doesn't mean that nothing sweet can ever cross your lips. It just means you have to indulge wisely.

How Much Sugar Can You Have?

The World Health Organization (WHO) recommends that you limit your intake of added sugars to no more than 10 percent of your calories. If you're an average-sized adult, that's somewhere around 50 grams of sugar, or the equivalent of 12 teaspoons or packets of granulated sugar. But they're not only talking about sugar that you might spoon into your coffee or onto your cereal. Added sugars refers to any sugar or concentrated sweetener (including honey and maple syrup) that you use in your own cooking or add at the table—as well as sugar that's been added to packaged and processed foods and beverages that you consume. You don't have to count the sugar that is naturally present in fruits, dairy products, and other whole foods.

Twelve packets of sugar might sound like a decent amount, but it adds up faster than you'd think. One 20-ounce bottle of soda and you've blown your budget for the day. Even if you don't drink soda, you might be surprised at how much sugar can hide in what seem like healthy foods. For example, a container of low-fat strawberry yogurt has 20 grams of added sugar. A low-fat bran muffin can have 45 grams of sugar. Even foods that don't taste particularly sweet, like wheat crackers or salad dressing, can have a teaspoon of added sugar per serving. It all adds up surprisingly quickly.

Added Sugar in Packaged Foods

The Nutrition Facts label on packaged foods tells you how many grams of sugar each serving contains. In foods that contain no dairy or fruit, assume that virtually all of the sugar listed on the label is an "added sugar." If the food contains dairy or fruit, it can be a little difficult to distinguish the added sugar from the naturally occurring sugars that you're not required to count toward your total. You may need to do a little detective work. For example, a container of plain yogurt contains 17 grams of sugar. A container of flavored yogurt that contains 37 grams of sugar therefore contains 20 grams of added sugar. For the recipes in this book, I've included the amount of total sugar as well as the amount of added sugar in each serving. You can also look up the nutrition facts for whole and packaged foods at Nutritiondata.com.

How Much Sugar Is in It?

1 teaspoon of white sugar = 4 grams
1 teaspoon of brown sugar (packed) = 4 grams
1 teaspoon of honey = 6 grams
1 teaspoon of maple syrup = 4 grams
1 scoop premium vanilla ice cream = 22 grams
1 scoop light vanilla ice cream = 17 grams
1 chocolate chip cookie = 10 grams
1 ounce dark chocolate = 10 grams

For the typical American, abiding by the WHO's limit on added sugar would mean cutting their sugar intake roughly in half. The killjoys at the American Heart Association (AHA) would like to lower the bar for added sugar even further, to just 5 percent of calories, or six packets of sugar per day. What accounts for the difference? The WHO's advice aims to keep healthy people healthy. The AHA's stricter guidelines are geared toward helping an already overweight, sedentary, and disease-ridden population reverse course.

Exercise dramatically improves your body's ability to metabolize sugar in a healthy way. So, I'm going to make a deal with you. Any day that you get at least thirty minutes of moderate intensity exercise, you've earned an extra bit of sweetness in your life. Enjoy up to

50 grams of added sugar, if you like. Otherwise, stick to the lower 25-gram limit. And, if you're trying to lose weight, I suggest that you limbo under the 25-gram bar until you've reached a healthy weight.

What about Chocolate?

As far as I'm concerned, as long as you stay within your budget, your sugar allowance is yours to spend however you want. But if you enjoy chocolate, indulging also offers some health benefits. Studies have found that eating chocolate can lower your blood pressure and your cholesterol, which of course is good for your heart health. But that's not all. Compounds in chocolate can increase your insulin sensitivity, which improves your body's ability to regulate your blood sugar and can help prevent type 2 diabetes. They also improve blood flow to the brain, which can make you smarter, or at least help you hang onto the intelligence you already have, as you get older. Chocolate also helps reduce inflammation, which helps prevent all kinds of diseases and just generally slows down the aging process. There's even research showing that eating chocolate on a regular basis can improve the texture and structure of your skin! And if all of that isn't enough, chocolate contains compounds that make you feel happier.

Most of the health benefits of chocolate are provided by compounds called flavanols and dark chocolate generally contains a lot more flavanols than milk chocolate. These days, dark chocolate is often marked with the percentage of cacao solids but higher percentages don't necessarily mean higher flavanol content. The type of cocoa bean, the region in which it was grown, and the processing methods are all factors. Most dark chocolate will have a decent amount of flavanols. See the box below for tips on chocolates that are particularly rich in these beneficial compounds.

What Kind of Chocolate Is Healthiest?

As with gourmet coffee, you can now buy gourmet dark chocolate with a pedigree that specifies what variety of beans it contains and where they were grown.

Region On average, cocoa beans grown in Ecuador, Colombia, and on the Ivory Coast have almost *twice* the flavanol content of beans from the Dominican Republic or Peru.

Variety The Amazon and Forestaro varieties are higher in flavanols than the Criollo variety.

Processing Flavanols are lost to a greater or lesser degree depending on how the beans are fermented, dried, and roasted. Some manufacturers, such as Callebaut and Mars, have developed special processing methods that minimize these losses. Acticoa (made by Callebaut) and CocoaVia (made by Mars) are two brands to look for.

Of course, in addition to all those healthy flavanols, chocolate also generally contains a good amount of sugar, fat, and calories. Despite all its benefits, chocolate—even dark chocolate—is a healthy food that you need to enjoy in moderation. Researchers estimate that eating just an ounce of dark chocolate every day is enough to get some positive benefit. But a single ounce of dark chocolate will set you back about 200 calories. Depending on the cacao percentage, it'll also cost you between 7 and 14 grams of added sugar. Although chocolate is good for you, you still need to fit the calories and the sugar into your daily budget.

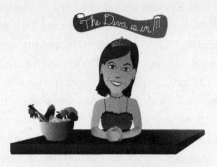

CHAPTER NINE

Curtain Calls

IN THE PREVIOUS five chapters, I've given you a sort of meal-by-meal template for how to make healthy choices throughout the day. Along the way, I've tried to answer as many frequently asked questions about diet and nutrition as I could without getting too sidetracked from that task. However, now that we've reached the end of our day, I realize that there are still some questions that I have not yet had a chance to address. I thought it might be easiest to tackle them here in a simple Q&A format that allows you to scan for the topics that interest you.

NUTRITIONAL SUPPLEMENTS

Should I Take a Multivitamin?

I always find this question a little tricky to answer. At one extreme, you have people who faithfully take their vitamins and then make horrendous diet choices day in and day out. I sometimes wonder whether taking a multivitamin gives folks a false sense of security and allows them to make a healthy diet less of a priority. For example, only one in three Americans manages to get the recommended servings of fruits and vegetables on a daily basis. Yet two out of three takes a multivitamin. If your diet is nutritionally deficient, getting nutrients from a pill is better than nothing but vitamin supplements are obviously no substitute for a healthy diet. What you eat will have a much bigger effect on your health than what vitamin pills you take.

At the other extreme you have people who make eating healthy nothing short of a religion. And then they gild the lily with two or three handfuls of high-potency nutritional supplements. I appreciate the enthusiasm. But they, too, are missing the point. More is not always better. For one thing, it's easy to overdo it. If you're taking several different supplements, for example, you can easily exceed the safe upper limits for certain nutrients. High doses of some nutrients can also interfere with the absorption of other nutrients.

Four Nutrients You Could Easily Be Overdoing

VITAMIN A—Vitamin A helps you see in the dark, fight off infections, and create red blood cells. The recommended amount is 3,000 IU for healthy adult men and a little less for adult women. (IU stands for International Units.) But many vitamin supplements—especially high-potency formulations—can contain as much as 5,000 IU. If you take a couple of different supplements, such as a multivitamin plus an immune-system booster, you could easily go over the safe upper limit of 10,000 IU. Signs of vitamin A overload include headaches, bone and joint pain, and itchy, peeling skin. Eventually, it can lead to liver damage. Check the label on any and all supplements that you take on a regular basis and make sure that the total amount of preformed Vitamin A, or retinol, doesn't exceed 2,500 IU per day. Supplements or foods that contain beta-carotene won't contribute to vitamin A overload because beta-carotene is converted to vitamin A only as needed.

FOLIC ACID—Folic acid helps you metabolize protein and synthesize DNA, protects against cancer and heart disease, and prevents serious birth defects. Healthy adults need 400 micrograms of folic acid a day; women need extra during pregnancy. Although it's important to get enough folic acid, more is not necessarily better. The main problem with getting too much folic acid from supplements is that it can mask B12 deficiency—and it's really important to diagnose and correct B12 deficiencies because they can lead to neurological damage. If you are pregnant or trying to get pregnant, your doctor will probably recommend a prenatal vitamin with the appropriate amount of folic acid. For everyone else, I suggest that you don't take more than 400 mcg per day of folic acid in supplement form. In addition, although folic acid generally protects against colon cancer, if you already have colon cancer, high doses of folic acid can feed tumor growth. If you have any history of colon cancer in your family, you'll want to be particularly careful about supplements— please check with your doctor for guidance. And, of course, everyone over fifty needs to be screened for colon cancer annually.

ZINC—Zinc is a critically important mineral, needed for thousands of cellular transactions in the body. Healthy adults need around 10 milligrams of zinc per day to meet their requirements and it turns out that that's about what people get from their diet, on average. But zinc is also a popular ingredient in dietary supplements. In addition to your multivitamins, you'll often find zinc in immune-boosting formulas, cold remedies, men's health, and prostate health formulas as well. If you're taking one or more of these on a daily basis, you could easily go over the recommended upper limit of 40 milligrams per day. One problem with taking too much zinc is that it interferes with your ability to absorb copper, another important nutrient. Copper deficiency can make you anemic as well as more susceptible to infection. Add up the zinc in any supplements you take on a regular basis and make sure it doesn't add up to more than 40 milligrams per day.

SELENIUM—Like all the others, selenium is an essential nutrient with important roles to play in your health. It's an antioxidant that helps make other antioxidants more potent, it helps protect against cancer, and it bolsters the immune system. The recommended intake for healthy adults is 55 micrograms per day and the average person gets about 100 micrograms from their diet, which is perfectly safe. But the safe upper limit for selenium is 400 micrograms per day, and if you're taking more than one vitamin supplement, you could easily be going over the limit. Add up the selenium in any supplements you take on a daily basis and make sure you're not getting more than 250 micrograms of selenium per day.

Get Your Nutrition from Foods, Not Pills

Study after study has found that taking a lot of extra nutritional supplements doesn't appear to make anyone any healthier. What does make people healthier is a balanced diet of nutritious, minimally processed foods—the kind of diet that I've described in this book.

THE QUICK AND DIRTY SECRET

Do the very best you can with your diet. Then, consider a basic one-a-day multivitamin to cover the gaps in a less-than-perfect diet—but leave it at that.

Should I Take a Calcium Supplement?

Fewer than half of Americans get the recommended amount of calcium from their diet. A lot of this could be solved by better eating habits. Vegetables can be a great source of calcium—especially kale, broccoli, Swiss chard, and collards. In fact, one cup of cooked collard greens has more calcium than a cup of milk. Plus, unlike most calcium supplements, vegetables are also rich in magnesium, vitamin K, and other nutrients that work with calcium to build strong bones. Five servings of vegetables can easily provide more than half of your daily calcium requirement. If you also drink milk or eat yogurt, each serving supplies about a third of your daily requirement. Beans, tofu, and sardines are other good sources. In other words, it's really not that hard to get the recommended amount of calcium from foods. If, however, you suspect that you're diet is falling short, you can take a supplement. Depending on how much calcium your diet provides, you may only need an additional 250 or 500 milligrams per day. Although it's important to get the recommended amount of calcium, there's no advantage to overdoing it.

Sadly, many women don't get serious about their calcium intake until they get into their thirties and forties—and their mothers begin to be diagnosed with osteoporosis. But you can't make up for the calcium that you failed to get earlier in life by doubling up later on. In fact, older women who take high doses of calcium from supplements may have an increased risk of heart attack.

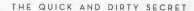

THE QUICK AND DIRTY SECRET

Take only as much calcium in supplement form as you need to cover the gap between your dietary intake and the recommended intake.

What about Vitamin D?

Vitamin D is very hot right now. Up until recently, vitamin D's big claim to fame was that it prevented rickets, a serious bone deformity that can affect kids and babies. Because vitamin D is not widespread in the food supply, health authorities in the United States decided back in 1932 that all milk should be fortified with vitamin D in order to prevent rickets. And that's pretty much the last anyone thought about it—until recently.

Over the last few years, researchers have noticed that people who have heart disease, diabetes, depression, various autoimmune diseases, osteoporosis, several types of cancer, and even obesity also seem to be low in vitamin D. And it turns out that lots of us are deficient in the vitamin. Seven out of ten American children, for example, are low in vitamin D. Vitamin D deficiency is also a particular concern in the elderly and those with dark skin, and everyone is at greater risk during the winter months.

The current recommended intake for vitamin D for adults is 200 to 400 IU. If you're over 70, it goes up to 600 IU. I think there's a fairly good chance that these recommendations will be raised within the next couple of years. The American Academy of Pediatrics has already increased its recommendation for children and adolescents from 200 to 400 IU.

A glass of milk has about 100 IU. A small serving of salmon has about 400 IU. Most multivitamins provide 200 to 400 IU and many calcium formulations now include vitamin D, as well. You can also meet your vitamin D needs by exposing your skin to the sun—without sunscreen.

You may have read that ten to fifteen minutes of sun per day will do the job. But it's a little more complicated than that. It all depends on where you are, how high you are, how much skin is exposed, how dark your skin is, the time of day, and the time of year. For example, in Washington, D.C., in August, you'd need just five minutes of sun at midday to top off your vitamin D stores. If you were two hundred miles north in New York City, you'd need an additional minute or so. If it were November in New York, you'd need about forty minutes. If it's November in New York and you have dark skin, you'd need two and a half hours. For most people, it's simpler just to take a supplement. Try to get at least 400 IU a day from foods and/or supplements, particularly in the winter or if you don't spend a lot of time outdoors without sunscreen.

Should I Take Fish Oil?

By now, almost everyone has heard about the omega-3 fatty acids and how important they are for your health. Omega-3s protect your heart and brain, lower your risk of cancer, heart attacks, and stroke, reduce inflammation, and have beneficial effects on your mood. In order for omega-3s to work their magic, there needs to be a balance between them and another family of essential fats called omega-6s, which have opposing but complementary functions. For most of us, though, our intake of these two families of fats is anything but balanced.

Fish are the richest sources of omega-3s, but some people don't care for fish and even those who like fish often don't eat it every day. Unlike the omega-3 fats, which are sort of few and far between in the food supply, omega-6 fatty acids are everywhere you turn. Vegetable oils such as corn, peanut, and soybean oils are very high in omega-6 fats. Because these oils are inexpensive, they are widely used in food processing and manufacturing. In the end, most of us get a lot of omega-6 in our diet, and not that much omega-3.

Taking a fish oil supplement is one way to solve the problem, and there's more hard evidence on the benefits of fish oil supplements than there is for almost any other dietary supplement. In fact, the demand for fish oil has gotten so huge that now there are serious concerns about the effects of overfishing. Another way to restore the balance is to reduce your intake of omega-6 fats.

How Can I Reduce My Omega-6 Intake?

- In the kitchen, use olive or canola oil instead of other vegetable oils.

- Read labels on processed foods and cut back on those that contain vegetable oils, including corn, soybean, peanut, sunflower, or safflower oils, especially if they contain more than a few grams of fat per serving.

- Sunflower seeds, sesame seeds, pine nuts, and peanuts are all rich in omega-6. You don't need to avoid them altogether but eating a lot of these foods will increase the amount of omega-3 you need to maintain a balance.

What about Flax?

Certain seeds, including flax, hemp, and chia, are also rich in omega-3s. But the kind of omega-3 found in these seeds isn't as potent as the form found in fish oil. Omega-3 actually refers to a whole family of fatty acids. At the top of the family tree is alphalinoleic acid, or ALA. It's the most common kind of omega-3, but it's also the least biologically active.

In order to get the most benefit from ALA, your body first has to convert it to other omega-3s like EPA and DHA. That conversion process isn't terribly efficient. Depending on the circumstances, only a small fraction of ALA may actually get converted into the turbo-powered EPA and DHA forms. The advantage of fish oil is that the fish have already done this conversion for you. Flax oil contains a whole bunch of ALA but almost no EPA or DHA. Fish oil, however, contains ALA but also lots of EPA and DHA.

So, flax doesn't necessarily have the same benefits as fish or fish oil. However, reducing your intake of omega-6 can make your body more efficient at converting ALA into EPA and DHA, making these vegetarian sources of omega-3 more valuable.

THE QUICK AND DIRTY SECRET

A fish oil supplement is fine. But you'll need less omega-3—and will get more benefit from vegetarian sources of omega-3—if you cut back on your omega-6 intake.

When's the Best Time to Take Your Vitamins?

Taking vitamins on an empty stomach can sometimes cause stomach upset. Taking them with food, which stimulates the release of digestive juices and enzymes, can also help you absorb the nutrients better. If your multivitamin contains iron and you also take a calcium supplement, it's a good idea to take them at different times. High doses of calcium, especially calcium carbonate, the form found in most supplements, can interfere with the absorption of iron. Try taking your multivitamin with breakfast or lunch and your calcium supplement at dinner or before bed. Taking calcium late in the day can also help you relax and fall asleep more easily.

NUTRITION AND EXERCISE

How Soon After Eating Should I Exercise?

You'll probably be most comfortable if you don't exercise on a full stomach. Working out too soon after a meal can cause acid reflux, side "stitches," or make you feel heavy or lethargic. As a general rule, wait one hour after a snack, two hours after a light to medium-sized meal, and at least three hours after a large meal before exercising. If you feel comfortable working out before breakfast, that's fine, too. (See "Will You Burn More Fat if You Exercise Before Breakfast?" page 112.)

What Should I Eat Before Exercising?

Ideally, you want to eat a normal-sized, healthy meal—you know, the kind with protein and vegetables—two to three hours before you exercise. If you're going to be exercising within the hour, it's best to focus on easily digested carbohydrates and keep your snack small. A banana, orange, or other piece of fruit; a small bagel, a container of yogurt, or a few graham crackers are all good snacks to eat before you exercise. You also want to be fully hydrated when you start exercising, so be sure to drink plenty of water ahead of time. Drinking sports drinks before exercising, however, really makes no sense.

When Should You Drink Sports Drinks?

It's important to stay hydrated and water is the ideal hydration beverage. If you are working out very hard, very long, or in very hot conditions, sports drinks like Gatorade, which contain electrolytes, are helpful. But water is really all you need for shorter or lower-intensity exercise. In fact, you can easily drink more calories than you burn by drinking sports drinks before, during, and after a moderate workout.

When Do You Need Energy Bars?

Bodies can easily store enough energy for about sixty minutes of sustained, high-intensity action. If you're exercising really hard for more than an hour or so, you can burn through your body's stash of stored fuel and run out of steam. During long workouts, eating (or drinking) some carbohydrates, which can be quickly converted to muscle energy, will allow you to exercise longer and harder. Just so we're clear, if you're reading *People* magazine on the treadmill for thirty minutes, you don't need an energy bar to get you through your workout. But if you're training with the U.S. swim team or biking across the Alps, you'll probably need to refuel during the workout. You don't want a protein bar or anything with a lot of fat or fiber in the middle of a workout because these are more work for the body to digest. In this situation, you want simple carbohydrates (otherwise known as sugar).

What Should I Eat After Exercising?

After a very vigorous or challenging work out, a "recovery meal" containing both protein and carbohydrate can help speed the repair and recovery of your muscles. But this is not the best time for a large protein-heavy meal. Research suggests that the ideal post work-out meal contains two to four times as much carbohydrate as protein and is relatively low in fat. There are sports drinks and powders formulated to provide the ideal proportions of nutrients. Ironically, low-fat chocolate milk performed just as well in trials. In fact, this is the one time that your body can handle—and even benefit from—a little extra sugar. So if you're hankering for something sweet, right after a workout is a good time to enjoy it.

How Soon Should I Eat After Exercising?

You'll get the most benefit from your recovery meal by eating it within thirty to sixty minutes. The timing is more critical if you're training very intensely, when even minute gains in performance can make a difference. And it doesn't have to be a full-sized meal—you can get just as much benefit from a recovery snack. If it's going to be a couple of hours before your next meal, plan to grab a small snack to bridge the gap.

DIET TRENDS

Are Low-carb Diets Healthier?

The term "low-carb diet" has many possible interpretations. To some, it means severely limiting all sources of carbohydrates—including fruits, dairy products, vegetables, and grains of any sort. Of course, when you eliminate all of these foods, you have to take nutritional supplements to supply most of your fiber, antioxidants, vitamins, and minerals—which strikes me as a sign of an imbalanced approach to nutrition. Low-carb dieters often experience very dramatic weight loss. But very few of them find either the diet or the weight loss to be sustainable over the long term.

To others, a low-carb diet means taking the top half of the bun off their hamburger or drinking low-carb beer. This type of "low-carb diet" is usually neither low-carb nor a diet, in the sense that it rarely leads to any weight loss.

In my opinion, the most useful variation on the low-carbohydrate approach is the one I've been advocating throughout this book: Simply limit your intake of refined flour, sugar, and things made with them. These foods are very easy to overeat, leading you to consume more calories than you need. For example, drinking sweetened beverages with a meal can add several hundred calories to your meal but doesn't make you feel any fuller or eat any less. A diet that is high in refined carbohydrates has a negative impact on blood-sugar levels, which affects appetite and energy levels and, ultimately, can lead to type 2 diabetes or even heart disease.

Finally, sweets, baked goods, breads, pasta, sweetened beverages, and so on, are also the least nourishing foods in the typical modern diet. You're certainly not missing out on anything you need by eliminating them from your diet.

Should I Adopt a Mediterranean Diet?

Back in the 1940s, epidemiologists—who are basically statisticians who focus on health—noticed that people from Crete seemed to live longer and stay healthier than people in northern Europe and North America—a lot healthier. So they took a closer look at how and what the people there ate—specifically, how their diet differed from the typical diet in less healthy regions. They noticed that the Cretans ate a lot less meat and poultry than other Westerners. When they did eat animal protein, it was more likely to be fish, which was not surprising, given that most people made their living fishing. They also ate a lot more fresh fruits, vegetables, and legumes and fewer processed, refined foods. They used a lot of olive oil. They tended to consume alcohol in moderation, mostly as red wine. This dietary pattern has come to be known as the Mediterranean diet.

When you compare the Mediterranean diet to the dietary guidelines put forth by the American Heart Association, you'll see that there are some interesting differences. For example, the Mediterranean diet is higher in fat than the AHA recommends. Despite that, the Mediterranean diet has become a popular and sanctioned alternative to the traditional low-fat heart-healthy diet.

Adopting the Mediterranean diet appears to reduce the risk of all kinds of diseases, including heart disease, cancer, Alzheimer's, Parkinson's, type 2 diabetes, and depression. It also appears to be a very effective way to lose weight and keep it off. Compared with people on low-fat and low-carb regimens, those following a Mediterranean diet lose just as much weight. More importantly, they tend to keep it off longer, perhaps because they find the diet satisfying and easy to stick with.

I think one of the reasons people seem to flourish on the Mediterranean diet is that it doesn't feel like a diet. It's a style of eating that focuses on positives (like eating more fresh vegetables) rather than negatives (like cutting out bread). Another thing I particularly like about the Mediterranean diet is that it defies the attempts of food manufacturers to reduce every diet trend into a new category of junk food. When low-fat diets were popular, manufacturers rushed to produce hundreds of new low-fat cookies and treats. They were low in fat but high in sugar, and it turned out to be pretty easy to gain weight eating low-fat foods.

Then, when low-carb diets came into fashion, the shelves were flooded with sugar- and carb-free meal replacement bars and drinks. They're low in carbs, all right, but four dozen unpronounceable chemicals listed as "ingredients" on the label makes me wonder if this really can be considered food. Instead of focusing on calories or fat or carbs, the Mediterranean diet emphasizes flavor, freshness, and the social and aesthetic pleasures of cooking and eating. It seems that good nutrition and healthy bodies tend to follow naturally.

Should Your Diet Be Based on Your Blood Type?

The different blood types—O, A, B, and AB—are genetic variations that appeared at various points in human evolution. Type O blood is thought to be the oldest surviving blood type, corresponding with the hunter-gatherer period. Type A blood appeared roughly twenty thousand years ago, coinciding with the dawn of primitive agriculture and the introduction of things like legumes and cereal grains to the human diet. The other blood types emerged even later, when humans were not only farming but also keeping livestock and consuming dairy products. They'd also begun to travel the globe, interbreed, and encounter a much wider variety of food species.

The basic idea behind the blood type diet is that you will be best nourished by the diet that was predominant when your blood type emerged. In other words, type O folks thrive on lots of meat and very few grains and dairy products. People with type A blood will be healthier eating a more plant-based diet. And the lucky types B and AB can pretty much eat anything!

It's a very interesting hypothesis but strong, substantive evidence for the benefits of eating a diet based on blood type is lacking. There are lots of anecdotal reports from people who experienced good results when following the blood-type diet but there haven't been any large, well-designed studies that have tested the hypothesis in a more scientific way.

The diet plans for the various blood types are all reasonably healthy. For example, none of them include Twinkies or French fries. (Apparently, the blood type that thrives on the typical modern diet has yet to emerge.) Obviously, anyone who eliminates junk food, refined sugar, and processed foods and replaces them with whole fruits and vegetables and lean protein is probably going to be a lot healthier. And that's what everyone following this diet will end up doing—regardless of their blood type. You'll also probably end up giving up a lot of healthy foods because they aren't "right" for your type. As long as you continue to eat other healthy foods, there's no harm in eliminating a few foods from your diet, but whether or not it's truly necessary is very much an open question.

Should You Eat a pH-Balancing Diet?

Some people believe that eating too many acid-forming foods causes our blood and/or tissues to become acidic and that this promotes disease. Every food you eat leaves a residue in the body after it is fully digested. That residue, or ash, is either acidic or alkaline. This has nothing to do with whether the food itself is acidic. For example, lemons are acidic, as you can tell by their pucker factor, but lemons leave an alkaline residue. The preferred terminology is that a lemon is an acidic food, but not an acid-*forming* food. In general, fruits and vegetables are alkaline-forming, whereas meats and grains are acid-forming.

It's absolutely true that maintaining the proper pH in your body is crucial—not just to staying healthy, but to staying alive at all. If your blood got even slightly too acidic or too alkaline and stayed that way for more than a few minutes, you'd be in a coma or worse. But what you eat actually has very little effect on the pH of your blood. Believe me, nature is not about to let your survival hinge on dietary discretion. We have several systems in place to maintain pH balance in our bodies, no matter what we eat.

What Does the pH of Your Urine Tell You?

Advocates of this theory often advise you to test the pH of your urine, using inexpensive pH sticks available at any drugstore. If you try this, you'll see that what you eat does change the pH of your urine. And to some, that is proof that the theory is valid. But the reason that your urine becomes more acidic when you eat acid-forming foods is so that your blood doesn't. The kidneys are one of the major ways that your body maintains a constant pH. In other words, worrying about the pH of your urine makes about as much sense as worrying about the dirt in your trash. Both are leaving the premises. The trash is carried out to the curb and any dirt it contains isn't going to make your house dirtier. Likewise, the pH level of the urine being flushed isn't making your body any more or less acidic.

A healthy body is able to maintain its pH no matter what you eat. However, if you eat too many acid-forming foods, that maintenance may have some costs. For example, one way that your body balances pH is to pull calcium from the bones. So eating too many acid-forming foods could theoretically promote bone loss. We don't have any research that directly or specifically links the acid/alkaline residue of the diet with health problems like osteoporosis. But there is indirect research that would seem to undermine this theory. For example, high-protein diets, which are presumably high in acid-forming foods, can increase bone loss—but only in people who are calcium deficient. In other words, if you are getting enough calcium and other minerals in your diet, you'll have more than enough to maintain your bone mass and buffer the effects of acid-forming foods.

In practice, a pH-balancing diet tends to be quite healthful. You end up eating lots of fruits and vegetables, which are high in anti-oxidants, vitamins, minerals, and fiber. And you cut out fried foods, refined grains, sugar, and most processed foods. Regardless of the pH aspect, that sounds to me like a good way to improve your health. In other words, I don't think anybody is going to get hurt following a pH-balanced diet, as long as the diet is otherwise balanced and nutritious. I just think that it's an unnecessarily complicated way to get to the same old punch line: Eat more vegetables, less junk, and nothing to excess.

STILL HAVE QUESTIONS?

There are so many fascinating aspects of diet and nutrition still to explore and I could go on forever. But at some point, this book must come to an end. If I've left you with burning questions unanswered (or a point you're dying to make), visit www.quickanddirtytips.com, where you'll find hundreds more nutrition questions (and answers) and lots of ways to participate in our ongoing conversation about food, diet, and nutrition. I hope you'll join me there.

In the meantime, get out there and eat something good for me!

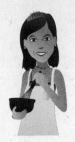

Nutrition Diva's Recipes

Apple Pie Oatmeal • 198

Warm Weather Oats • 199

Leftover Vegetable Frittata • 200

Breakfast Burrito • 201

Salmon and Rotini Salad • 202

Tofu Salad with Nutritional Yeast • 203

Asian-style Broccoli Salad • 204

Curried Tuna Salad • 205

Best Fruit and Nut Bars • 206

Tomatillo Guacamole • 207

Goat Cheese Spread with Figs • 208

Silken Asparagus Soup • 209

Sweet Potato and Cauliflower Curry • 210

Roasted Cauliflower • 211

Braised Fennel • 212

Tender Kale • 213

Quinoa Salad with Pecans and Cranberries • 214

Penne with Sautéed Chard • 215

Crunchy Sesame Flax Chicken • 216

Moroccan Sliders • 217

Ras El Hanout (Moroccan Spice Mixture) • 218

Louisiana Red Beans and Rice • 219

Chili con Cocoa • 220

Fish Soup • 221

APPLE PIE OATMEAL

Serves 1

¾ cup water

⅓ cup old-fashioned rolled oats or rolled whole grains

½ small apple, diced

¼ teaspoon apple (or pumpkin) pie seasoning or cinnamon

Pinch of salt

2 tablespoons chopped walnuts

Honey, maple syrup, or other sweetener, to taste

1. Combine water, oats or grains, apple, spices, and salt in saucepan and cook over low heat, stirring occasionally, until creamy, about 6–8 minutes.

2. Spoon into individual bowls, sprinkle with nuts, and top (sparingly) with honey, maple syrup, or another sweetener.

TIP: You'll need less sweetener if you drizzle or sprinkle it on top rather than stirring it in.

NUTRITION INFORMATION (PER SERVING), NOT INCLUDING ADDED SWEETENER: *Calories 245, Carbohydrates 33g, Fiber 6g, Sugar 9g (added sugars, 0g), Protein 6g, Fat 20g*

WARM WEATHER OATS

Serves 1

This make-ahead breakfast is a great timesaver on busy mornings. It's also a nice way to enjoy the goodness of oatmeal, even when the weather is too warm for hot cereal.

    ¼ cup rolled oats
    ¼ cup fresh or frozen wild blueberries (or other seasonal fruit)
    ⅓ cup plain yogurt
    ⅓ cup water
    2 tablespoons almonds, coarsely chopped
    Honey, maple syrup, or other sweetener to taste

1. Place oats, fruit, yogurt, and water in bowl, stir, and refrigerate overnight.
2. Before serving, add nuts, and top (sparingly) with sweetener.

TIP: You'll need less sweetener if you drizzle or sprinkle it on top rather than stir it in.

NUTRITION INFORMATION (PER SERVING), NOT INCLUDING ADDED SWEETENER: *Calories 225, Carbohydrates 28g, Fiber 5g, Sugar 7g (added sugar 0g), Protein 10g, Fat 9g*

LEFTOVER VEGETABLE FRITTATA

Serves 4

A veggie-stuffed frittata is a great way to get an extra serving of vegetables into your day. Using leftover vegetables makes it quick and easy.

> 6 eggs
>
> Dash Worcestershire sauce
>
> Salt and pepper, to taste
>
> 2 cups leftover cooked vegetables, such as broccoli, zucchini, asparagus, or spinach
>
> ½ cup crumbled feta, goat cheese, or shredded hard cheese

1. Preheat broiler
2. In medium bowl, whisk eggs, Worcestershire sauce, salt and pepper until blended.
3. Spray 10-inch oven-proof skillet with nonstick spray and heat over medium heat.
4. Add vegetables to skillet and sauté briefly. Spread evenly around skillet. Pour egg mixture into pan. Use tongs to redistribute veggies, if necessary, and press them down into the eggs.
5. Cook over medium heat until edges are set (about 5 minutes).
6. Sprinkle with cheese and put skillet into broiler until puffed and brown (another 3 to 5 minutes). Remove carefully with pot holder and serve warm.

NUTRITION INFORMATION (PER SERVING):
Calories 184, Carbohydrates 7g, Fiber 3g, Sugar 2g (added sugar 0g), Protein 14g, Fat 12g.

BREAKFAST BURRITO

Serves 1

¼ cup refried beans

one 8-inch flour tortilla

¼ cup grated cheese (such as cheddar or Colby)

1 egg

Cilantro (optional)

Salsa and reduced fat sour cream

1. Preheat broiler or toaster oven. Spread refried beans in center of each tortilla. Top with half the cheese.

2. Spray skillet with nonstick spray and heat over medium heat. Fry eggs, breaking yolk if desired. Use a spatula to transfer fried egg to tortilla and roll into loose cigar.

3. Place rolled tortillas seam side down on foil-lined broiler tray and sprinkle with remaining cheese. Broil until cheese is bubbly and tortillas are crisp at edges. Sprinkle with chopped cilantro if desired, and serve with salsa and reduced-fat sour cream.

NUTRITION INFORMATION (PER SERVING):

Calories 412, Carbohydrates 37g, Fiber 3g, Sugar 1g (added sugar 0g), Protein 22g, Fat 20g

SALMON AND ROTINI SALAD

Serves 4

The dressing for this salad is simple to allow the flavors of the other ingredients to shine. Fresh herbs are nonnegotiable here, but you can substitute 2 tablespoons of fresh dill for the parsley.

- 4 ounces rotini pasta, or 2 cups leftover cooked pasta
- 2 cans of salmon, or leftover cooked salmon
- 3 tablespoons reduced fat mayonnaise
- 1½ tablespoons lemon juice
- ¼ teaspoon ground pepper
- 1 large red pepper, diced (about 1 cup)
- ½ cup diced onion
- ½ cup diced celery
- 1 small bunch flat leaf Italian parsley, finely chopped (about ¼ cup packed)
- Salt, to taste

1. Cook pasta according to package directions. Drain and cool.
2. Drain salmon and separate into bite-sized pieces using a fork or your fingers.
3. Whisk mayonnaise, lemon juice, and pepper together in large bowl.
4. Add pasta, salmon, red pepper, onion, celery, and parsley. Toss to combine and season to taste with salt.

NUTRITION INFORMATION (PER SERVING):
Calories 225, Carbohydrates 27g, Fiber 4g, Sugar 3g (added sugars, 0g), Protein 16g, Fat 7g.

TOFU SALAD WITH NUTRITIONAL YEAST

Serves 4

I used to think of this as a mock egg salad until I realized that I like it much better than regular egg salad! Great on crackers or as a sandwich or wrap filling.

> 1 package extra-firm regular (not silken) tofu
> 1 medium carrot, grated
> 3 tablespoons light mayonnaise
> 3 tablespoons nutritional yeast flakes (not brewer's yeast)
> Garlic salt, to taste

1. Wrap tofu in several thicknesses of paper towels and squeeze to remove excess moisture.
2. Mash tofu with fork in medium bowl.
3. Add rest of ingredients and combine. Adjust seasoning to taste.

NUTRITION INFORMATION (PER SERVING):
Calories 164, Carbohydrates 8g, Fiber 4g, Sugars 2g (added sugar 0g), Protein 14g, Fat 9g.

ASIAN-STYLE BROCCOLI SALAD

Serves 4

2 bunches fresh broccoli (about 6 cups chopped)

¼ cup blanched almonds, slivered or chopped

2 tablespoons seasoned rice vinegar

1 tablespoon honey

2 teaspoons minced fresh ginger

1 teaspoon soy sauce

1 teaspoon toasted sesame oil

½ red or vidalia onion, diced

1. Separate broccoli into florets and chop the top 2 inches of stem into 1-inch cubes. Place broccoli in briskly boiling, salted water and boil until just tender and crisp, about 2½ to 3 minutes. Immediately drain broccoli and plunge into cold water to stop the cooking process. Drain well.

2. Toast almonds in a dry skillet over medium heat until fragrant and golden. Shake often and watch carefully to prevent burning. Set aside.

3. In a large bowl, whisk together seasoned rice vinegar, honey, ginger, soy sauce, and sesame oil. Add broccoli and chopped onion to dressing and toss well.

4. Just before serving, add almonds to salad and toss lightly. Serve salad at room temperature or slightly chilled.

NUTRITION INFORMATION (PER SERVING):
Calories 131, Carbohydrates 19g, Fiber 6g, Sugar 12g (added sugar 7g) , Protein 7g, Fat 5g.

CURRIED TUNA SALAD

Serves 4

Tired of the same old tuna salad? Try this sophisticated grown-up version instead. The curry powder gives it a natural anti-inflammatory kick!

1 can (6 oz) tuna, drained

¼ cup grated carrot

3 tablespoons light mayonnaise

2 tablespoons pine nuts

2 tablespoons golden raisins

2 teaspoons curry powder

1. Drain tuna and mash with fork.
2. Add remaining ingredients and combine well.

NUTRITION INFORMATION (PER SERVING):
Calories 143, Carbohydrate 6g, Fiber 1g, Sugar 4g (added sugar, 0g), Protein 12g, Fat 7g.

BEST FRUIT AND NUT BARS

Makes 12 bars

Better than any store-bought energy bars, these are great for breakfast-on-the-go, brown-bag lunches, and snacks. Make a batch on the weekend to get you through the work week.

> ½ cup whole flaxseed (or ⅔ cup ground flax)
>
> ½ cup peanut butter
>
> ⅓ cup honey
>
> Pinch salt (two pinches if peanut butter is unsalted)
>
> ⅓ cup water
>
> ⅔ cup dried fruits (raisins, cranberries, chopped apricots, etc.)
>
> ⅔ cup nuts or seeds (sunflower, pumpkin, chopped almonds, etc.)

1. Preheat oven to 325.
2. Grind whole flaxseed in a coffee or spice grinder. Combine with peanut butter, honey, salt, and water in large bowl and stir to combine.
3. Add dried fruits, nuts, and seeds in whatever combination you like. Batter will be very stiff.
4. Spray 12-cup muffin tin with nonstick spray and divide batter evenly into cups. Use damp fingers to press batter into cups and flatten tops.
5. Bake 25 to 30 minutes until tops are dry and edges are a deep, toasty brown (bars will not rise). Cool completely and store in airtight container for up to two weeks.

NUTRITION INFORMATION (PER SERVING):
Calories 200, Carbohydrates 19g, Fiber 4g, Sugar 13g (added sugar 9g) Protein 6g, Fat 12g.

TOMATILLO GUACAMOLE

Serves 4

4 tomatillos

½ - 1 jalapeno pepper (to taste), membranes and seeds removed.

1 small clove garlic

¼ cup cilantro leaves

1 ripe avocado

Juice from half a lime (about 1 tablespoon)

1. Remove husks from tomatillos and rinse to remove any sticky residue.
2. Pulse tomatillos, jalapeno, garlic, and cilantro in mini food processor until finely minced.
3. Mash avocado in bowl with lime juice.
4. Stir in tomatillo mixture and chill 1 hour before serving.
5. Makes about 1 cup.

NUTRITION INFORMATION (PER SERVING):
Calories 97, Carbohydrate 8g, Fiber 4g, Sugar 2g, (added sugar 0g), Protein 1g.

GOAT CHEESE SPREAD
WITH FIGS AND BLACK PEPPER

Serves 6

This elegant and sophisticated spreads requires a few high-end ingredients but takes just seconds to whip up. Make it for your next fancy dinner or cocktail party—or anytime you're in the mood for a gourmet treat.

> 4 ounces reduced-fat goat cheese
> 2 ounces black mission figs (about 6), finely chopped
> 1 tablespoon argan oil (available in gourmet stores) or
> toasted walnut oil
> 2 teaspoons honey
> 3/4 teaspoon coarsely cracked black pepper

1. Combine all ingredients and stir briskly with a wooden spoon (or beat at low speed in electric mixer) until well combined and fluffy. Serve with green apple slices or crackers. Makes about 3/4 cup.

NUTRITION INFORMATION (PER SERVING):
Calories 88, Carbohydrates 7g, Fiber 1g, Sugar 6g (added sugar 2g), Protein 4g, Fat 5g.

SILKEN ASPARAGUS SOUP

Serves 4

You'd never guess that this elegantly creamy soup is completely dairy-free!
For a more substantial dish, add 3 or 4 peeled cooked shrimp to each bowl
before serving. The hot soup will warm the shrimp without overcooking them.

   1 tablespoon olive oil

   2 shallots or 1 medium onion, chopped

   1 pound very slender asparagus spears, tough ends discarded

   2 14-ounce cans low sodium chicken stock, or 3½ cups
      homemade stock

   1 bay leaf

   1 spring fresh thyme (or ¼ teaspoon dried thyme)

   1 teaspoon sea salt

   ½ teaspoon ground pepper

   6 ounces (½ package) extra-firm silken tofu

1. Heat oil in large pot over medium low heat and add shallots or
onion, cooking until softened.

2. Break the top 2 inches off of each asparagus spear and set aside.
Break remaining stem into 2-inch pieces.

3. Add stock, bay leaf, thyme, salt, pepper, and asparagus stems to
onion and simmer over low heat about 20 to 25 minutes, until asparagus stems are quite tender. Remove bay leaf.

4. Transfer soup to blender and add tofu. Blend until perfectly
smooth (work in two batches if necessary).

5. Return pureed soup to pot and add a bit of hot water if needed
to correct consistency and salt, if needed. Add asparagus tips and
simmer over low heat 5 to 10 minutes until asparagus spears are just
tender. (If you are working with thicker asparagus, steam tips briefly
over boiling water before adding to soup.)

NUTRITION INFORMATION (PER SERVING):
*Calories 155, Carbohydrates 14g, Fiber 2g, Sugar 6g (added sugar 0g),
Protein 11g, Fat 7g.*

SWEET POTATO AND CAULIFLOWER CURRY

Serves 6

Traditional Indian cookery typically involves a long list of exotic spices. This variation involves fewer ingredients and steps but is every bit as exotic and colorful.

  3 tablespoons canola oil

  2 onions, finely chopped

  1 medium (5- to 6-inch) sweet potato, diced

  1 head cauliflower, broken into small florets

  1 teaspoon minced ginger

  2 tablespoons curry powder

  1 teaspoon salt

  1 cup stock or water

  3 tablespoons plain yogurt

  1 cup frozen peas

  2 tomatoes, quartered

1. Heat oil in large pan and saute onions over medium heat until translucent.

2. Add sweet potato, cauliflower, ginger, curry powder, and salt. Stir to combine and cook 5 minutes.

3. Stir in stock or water and yogurt. Cover and simmer over low heat for 20 minutes.

4. Add peas and tomatoes and cook 10 minutes or until all vegetables are tender.

NUTRITION INFORMATION (PER SERVING):
Calories 148, Carbohydrate 18g, Fiber 5g, Sugar 7g (added sugar 0g), Protein 5g, Fat 7g.

ROASTED CAULIFLOWER

Serves 4

Even those who don't think they like cauliflower will go for this! Use the same method to roast halved Brussels sprouts or cubed butternut squash.

    3 tablespoons 100% olive oil
    1-2 cloves mashed garlic (optional)
    1 medium head cauliflower
    Salt and pepper to taste

1. Preheat oven to 400 degrees and place oven rack in lower third of oven.
2. Place olive oil in large bowl. Put garlic (if using) through a garlic press and add to oil.
3. Break cauliflower into small florets and toss with olive oil to coat. Arrange in single layer on cookie sheet and season with salt and pepper.
4. Roast for 20-25 minutes, stirring once after 15 minutes. Cauliflower should be well browned.

NUTRITION INFORMATION (PER SERVING):
Calories 128, Carbohydrates 6g, Fiber 4g, Sugar 3g (added sugar 0g), Protein 3g, Fat 10g.

BRAISED FENNEL

Serves 2

Braised fennel makes a terrific side dish for baked or grilled fish.

1 tablespoon canola oil

1 teaspoon butter

1 large fennel bulb, cored and cut into thin strips

1 tablespoon balsamic vinegar

¼ cup chicken stock or water

1 teaspoon honey

¼ teaspoon salt

¼ teaspoon pepper

1. Heat oil and butter in skillet and add fennel.
2. Cook over medium heat, stirring frequently, about ten minutes, until lightly browned
3. Add vinegar to fennel and scrape up any browned bits from pan.
4. Add chicken stock or water to pan, cover and cook an additional 15 minutes, or until tender.
5. Drizzle with honey and season with salt and pepper.

NUTRITION INFORMATION (PER SERVING):
Calories 145, Carbohydrates 14g, Fiber 4g, Sugar 5g (Added sugar 3g), Protein 2g, Fat 10g.

TENDER KALE

Serves 4

Kale requires longer cooking times than chard or spinach. This method gives you tender succulent greens and minimizes nutrient losses.

  1 large bunch kale, washed
  2 tablespoons olive oil
  2 shallots or 1 small onion, thinly sliced
  ⅓ cup water or chicken stock
  1 tablespoon balsamic vinegar
  Salt and pepper, to taste

1. Coarsely chop kale, discarding tough stems.
2. Heat olive oil in large skillet until shimmering and add shallots. Sauté over medium heat until softened.
3. Add kale to pan, moving it around with tongs to wilt it evenly.
4. When kale is wilted, add stock, tightly cover skillet and turn heat to low. Simmer until liquid is absorbed, about 10–15 minutes. If kale is not yet tender, add a few more tablespoons of liquid and continue to simmer gently.
5. When kale is tender but still bright green, remove the lid and turn up the heat to cook off any remaining liquid. Add balsamic vinegar and salt and pepper, to taste.

NUTRITION INFORMATION (PER SERVING):
Calories 137, Carbohydrates 16g, Fiber 3g, Sugar 1g (added sugar 0g), Protein 5g, Fat 8g.

QUINOA SALAD
WITH PECANS AND CRANBERRIES

Serves 4

For the best flavor, serve salad at room temperature or slightly chilled. This makes a great salad for potlucks and picnics.

> 1 cup quinoa
> 1½ cup water
> ½ teaspoon salt
> ¼ cup chopped pecans (or walnuts)
> 3 tablespoons seasoned rice vinegar
> 1 tablespoon walnut oil
> ⅓ cup dried cranberries
> Salt and pepper to taste

1. Place quinoa in a sieve and rinse thoroughly under running water to remove the grain's bitter coating.
2. Put quinoa, water, and salt in saucepan and bring to a boil. Reduce heat to low, cover, and cook until water is absorbed, about 15 minutes (check frequently). When water is absorbed, test quinoa for tenderness. If it is not yet tender, add a bit more water and cook until absorbed. Remove from heat and allow to cool in the pan, still covered.
3. While quinoa is cooling, toast pecans briefly in a dry skillet over medium low heat, just until fragrant.
4. Place seasoned vinegar in large mixing bowl and add walnut oil in a thin stream while whisking briskly.
5. Add quinoa, pecans, and cranberries and toss to combine. Season with salt and pepper to taste.

NUTRITION INFORMATION (PER SERVING):
Calories 282, Carbohydrates 40g, Fiber 4g, Sugar 11g (added sugar 11g), Protein 7g, Fat 11g.

PENNE WITH SAUTÉED CHARD

Serves 4

You can substitute a large bag of spinach for the chard in this recipe. Sautéed chard (without the pasta) also makes a delicious vegetable side dish.

> 4 ounces dry pasta
> 2 large bunches Swiss chard, washed
> 4 tablespoons olive oil
> 3 cloves garlic
> ¼ teaspoon ground black pepper
> Salt, to taste

1. Boil penne in plenty of salted water, until tender. Drain and return to pot.
2. Coarsely chop the chard, discarding large ribs.
3. Heat olive oil in large skillet and add garlic, sautéing briefly until golden. Add chard to skillet and saute until tender, about 5 minutes. (Use tongs to move the chard around the skillet until it is uniformly wilted.)
4. Season with pepper and salt, to taste.
5. Portion pasta into bowls and top with chard. Drizzle with additional olive oil if desired

NUTRITION INFORMATION (PER SERVING):
Calories 242, Carbohydrates 25g, Fiber 4, Sugar 1g (added sugar 0g), Protein 6g, Fat 14g.

CRUNCHY SESAME FLAX CHICKEN

Serves 4

Try this next time you get a craving for decadent fried chicken. Instead of excess fat and calories, you get the goodness of wheat germ and flaxseed.

½ cup low-sodium soy sauce

1 clove garlic, crushed

4 uncooked chicken breasts, skins removed

¼ cup flaxseeds

¼ cup bread crumbs

2 tablespoons wheat germ

2 tablespoons sesame seeds

2 tablespoons dried parsley

1 tablespoon canola oil

1. Combine soy sauce and garlic in a small dish and marinate raw chicken pieces for 10–20 minutes, turning once.

2. Grind flaxseed in blender or coffee grinder and mix with bread crumbs, wheat germ, sesame seeds, and parsley.

3. Remove chicken from soy sauce and roll in breading mixture. Lay on greased baking sheet. Drizzle with oil. Bake 25–35 minutes at 400 degrees, until juices run clear when chicken is pierced.

NUTRITION INFORMATION (PER SERVING):
Calories 291, Carbohydrate 11g, Fiber 4g, Sugar 1g (added sugar 0g), Protein 31g, Fat 14g.

MOROCCAN SLIDERS

Serves 4

Fragrant spices contain antioxidants that block the formation of harmful chemicals when these little burgers are grilled. In the summer, I like to serve these with a simple salad made of sliced cucumbers, a splash of seasoned rice vinegar, and a pinch of dill.

> 1 pound lean ground beef or bison
> 1 tablespoon Morrocan spice mixture (recipe follows)

1. Prepare charcoal or preheat gas grill.
2. Mix meat and spices. Form into 8 miniature burgers, about two inches in diameter.
3. Grill burgers 3-4 minutes per side.

NUTRITION INFORMATION (PER SERVING):
Calories 152, Carbohydrates 0g, Fiber 0g, Sugar 0g, Protein 22g, Fat 7g.

RAS EL HANOUT (MOROCCAN SPICE MIXTURE)

Makes about 2 tablespoons

1 teaspoon cumin

1 teaspoon ginger

3/4 teaspoon salt

3/4 teaspoon black pepper

1/2 teaspoon ground cinnamon

1/2 teaspoon ground coriander

1/2 teaspoon cayenne pepper

1/2 teaspoon allspice

1/4 teaspoon ground cloves

1. Blend all the spices in a small bowl and store in an airtight container. Use to season roasted or grilled meats, vegetable stews, rice, or couscous.

LOUISIANA RED BEANS AND RICE

Serves 4

This dish tastes even better the next day, so plan to take some for lunch.

1 cup diced onion

½ cup diced celery

½ cup diced green pepper

2 tablespoons extra-virgin olive oil

2 cloves garlic, mashed

3 cups cooked red beans (or two 15-ounce cans of small red beans or dark red kidney beans, drained)

3 cups water

2 teaspoons Worcestershire sauce

1 teaspoon salt (or reduced sodium salt)

½ teaspoon cayenne pepper

¼ teaspoon cumin

¼ teaspoon dried thyme

¼ teaspoon ground black pepper

2 cups cooked brown rice

Louisiana hot sauce (optional)

1. Sauté onion, celery, and green pepper in olive oil over medium heat for about 10 minutes. Add garlic and sauté two more minutes.

2. Add the rest of the ingredients (except for rice) and simmer for 30–40 minutes. Stir occasionally, more frequently toward the end of the cooking time. As you stir, mash some of the beans with the back of your spoon to thicken the mixture.

3. Place ½ cup cooked rice in a bowl. Ladle one cup of bean mixture over the top. Add a dash of Louisiana hot sauce, if desired.

NUTRITION INFORMATION (PER SERVING):
Calories: 353, Carbohydrates 58g, Fiber 15g, Sugar 3g (added sugar 0g), Protein 15g, Fat 7g.

CHILI CON COCOA

Serves 6

Cocoa powder adds depth to the flavor, plus all the healthy benefits of dark chocolate with none of the sugar! This is another one that's even better the next day and will be great to pack for lunch.

2 tablespoons olive or canola oil

1 large onion, diced

1 pound lean ground beef or bison

3 tablespoons chili powder

1 tablespoon cocoa powder (not "dutched")

1 teaspoon salt

3 15-ounce cans small white (northern) beans, drained
    (or 4–5 cups cooked white beans)

3 14-ounce cans crushed tomatoes

1 cup water

1. Heat oil in bottom of large pan or Dutch oven until hot, but not smoking. Add onion and cook over medium heat until softened, about 5 minutes.

2. Add meat and stir to brown evenly. When meat is fully browned, stir in chili powder, cocoa powder, and salt and cook for 2 minutes.

3. Add beans, tomatoes, and 1 cup water. Turn heat to low (but do not cover) and simmer 45–60 minutes.

NUTRITION INFORMATION (PER SERVING):
Calories 450, Carbohydrates 54g, Fiber 20g, Sugar 1g (added sugar 0g), Protein 31g, Fat 14g

FISH SOUP

Serves 4

An elegant alternative to thick, heavy chowders, this soup is light enough to serve in warm weather.

1 large leek
1 tablespoon canola oil
1 tablespoon butter
2 medium boiling potatoes (or 6 small red potatoes), cubed
2 1/2 cups water
1/2 teaspoon salt
1/4 teaspoon black pepper
1 pound frozen white fish (haddock or cod), thawed
1 cup evaporated milk
Fresh parsley, chopped

1. Remove green tops from leeks and discard. Wash leeks thoroughly to remove any sand and chop finely.
2. Heat oil and butter in large pot or Dutch oven. Add leek and sauté over low heat until tender and golden, about 8 minutes.
3. Add potatoes, water, salt, and pepper and bring to a boil. Reduce heat to low and simmer 8–10 minutes.
4. Add fish and simmer another 10 minutes. Stir in evaporated milk and heat to serving temperature. Garnish with chopped parsley.

NUTRITION INFORMATION (PER SERVING):
Calories 301, Carbohydrates 22g, Fiber 2g, Sugar 7g (added sugar, 0g), Protein 27g, Fat 12g.

SAMPLE MEAL PLANS

To give you an idea how the advice in this book looks in practice, here are some examples of healthy meal plans for various types of eaters. For more details about putting together healthy meals, please refer to the individual chapters in Part Two.

The Three-square 2000

breakfast	Breakfast Burrito (recipe on page 201) fruit salad or piece of fruit
lunch	turkey, Swiss, and avocado sandwich on whole-grain bread Asian Broccoli Salad (recipe on page 204) or green salad
snack	Fruit and Nut Bar (recipe on page 206) or quarter cup of dried fruit and nut trail mix
dinner	Crunchy Sesame Flax Chicken (recipe on page 216) or broiled chicken breast ½ baked acorn squash brushed with butter and maple syrup roasted green beans

This meal plan provides about 2000 calories in three meals (plus one snack).

The Lightweight 1600

breakfast	Leftover Vegetable Frittata (recipe on page 200) or scrambled eggs and salsa 1 piece whole-grain toast with butter
lunch	Curried Tuna Salad (recipe on page 205) or tuna salad on bed of greens with cherry tomatoes whole-grain bread stick or cracker
snack	small serving of cheese seasonal fruit
dinner	pork tenderloin sautéed spinach or Swiss chard Roasted Cauliflower (recipe on page 211)

This meal plan is provides about 1600 calories, for those who are smaller, older, and/or less active.

The Power House 2400

breakfast	three-egg omelet with smoked salmon and vegetables or smoothie made with yogurt, banana, and peanut butter whole grain English muffin with butter
lunch	two fish tacos with shredded cabbage and salsa side of beans and rice
snack	cottage cheese and fruit
dinner	grilled flank steak Quinoa Salad with Pecans and Cranberries (recipe on page 214) or rice pilaf steamed broccoli

This meal plan provides about 2400 calories and is higher in protein, for those who are larger, younger, and/or more active.

The Snacker 2000

breakfast	oatmeal with honey and chopped walnuts
morning snack	latte apple
lunch	bowl of minestrone soup whole grain roll hard-boiled egg
afternoon snack	green salad with blue cheese and pear or raw vegetables and hummus
dinner	grilled fish Braised Fennel (see recipe on page 212) or Tender Kale (see recipe on page 213) steamed rice or quinoa
evening snack	baked sweet potato cottage cheese or yogurt

This meal plan provides about 2000 calories, divided into six small meals.

The Vegivore 1800

breakfast	Apple Pie Oatmeal (recipe on page 198), soymilk latte
lunch	Tofu Salad with Nutritional Yeast on whole grain bread or crackers (recipe on page 203) cucumber salad seasonal fruit
snack	grapefruit and avocado salad
dinner	Louisiana Red Beans and Rice (recipe on page 219) tossed salad with oil and vinegar baked apple

This meal plan provides about 1800 calories and contains no meat, poultry, fish, eggs, or dairy products.

The Decadent Diva 2000

breakfast in bed	low-fat Greek yogurt topped with berries, chopped almonds, and drizzle of honey
mid-morning snack	half a whole grain bagel with cream cheese and smoked salmon
late lunch	Silken Asparagus Soup (recipe on page 209) sliced cucumbers with Goat Cheese spread with Figs and Black Pepper (recipe on page 208) square of dark chocolate
dining in	Moroccan Sliders (recipe on page 217) on whole wheat pita grilled vegetables cucumber salad
evening indulgence	glass of wine buttered popcorn

This meal plan provides about 2000 calories and includes a glass of wine and a serving of chocolate.

Here's a cheat sheet to take to the grocery store, with summaries and reminders of the tips in Part One. For a printer-friendly shopping list and guide, visit www.nutritiondivabook.com.

VEGETABLES	FRUIT
Aim for two and a half cups per day per person.	Aim for two cups per day per person.
Go for variety: • Green (lettuce, spinach, kale, Swiss chard, beet and mustard greens, etc.) • Red/orange (tomatoes, carrots, sweet potatoes, winter squash, red peppers) • Cruciferous (cabbage, broccoli, cauliflower, Brussels sprouts) • Pods (peas, green beans, snowpeas, etc.) • Stinkers (onions, scallions, shallots, garlic)	Particularly nutritious: • Apricots (fresh) • Berries (all kinds) • Cantaloupe • Cherries • Citrus • Grapes (especially red or purple) • Kiwi • Pomegranate
High in pesticide residues: • Bell peppers • Celery • Spinach • Lettuce • Potatoes	High in pesticide residues: • Peaches • Apples • Nectarines • Strawberries • Cherries • Pears • Imported grapes

MILK	NON-DAIRY MILK ALTERNATIVES
Nutritionally speaking, organic milk is comparable to conventional milk. But buying organic reduces the use of antibiotics in livestock, which is definitely better for you and the environment.	Dairy-free milk should contain no more than 12g sugar and 100mg sodium per serving. **Higher in protein**: soy milk **Lower in sugar/calories**: almond milk **Higher in fiber**: soy milk, oat milk **Higher in omega-3**: hemp

BUTTER OR MARGARINE	SOUR CREAM, CREAM CHEESE, ETC.
Avoid spreads made with hydrogenated and/or esterified oils.	Choose low or reduced fat products to save calories but avoid fat-free products that contain a lot of artificial ingredients and additives.

CHEESE	YOGURT
Higher in protein and calcium: Gruyere, Parmesan, Gouda, cottage cheese **Lower in fat and calories**: part-skim ricotta, mozzarella, feta, goat, cottage cheese **Lower in sodium**: Camembert, Swiss **Note:** If you're watching sodium, avoid cottage cheese, blue cheese, gouda, feta, and parmesan.	Plain, unsweetened yogurt is best. Look for products labeled "Live and active cultures." Lemon, vanilla, and coffee-flavored yogurts have about 25% less sugar than most fruit-flavored yogurts.

EGGS	JUICE
Most healthy adults can eat a dozen or so eggs a week without adverse effects on their cholesterol levels or heart disease risk.	Limit juice to one serving a day. Citrus, pomegranate, and grape juice are the most nutritious choices.

FRESH MEAT	DELI
Boneless cuts: Allow 4 ounces per portion Cuts with bones: Allow 6 to 8 ounces per portion (Portion = 3 ounces cooked meat) **Best choices** **Beef:** tenderloin, strip steak, top sirloin, T-bone, flank steak, London broil **Bison:** all **Lamb:** loin chops, leg of lamb **Pork:** tenderloin, loin roast **Poultry:** skinless breast	1 pound = 16 medium-thick slices or 25 to 30 thin slices **Best choices** Lower-sodium roast beef, chicken, or turkey **Note:** Pregnant women, small children, and those who eat cured meats more than once or twice a week should buy nitrite-free products.

FRESH MEAT	DELI
Budget friendly: ground beef, bison, chicken, or turkey (90% lean), chuck roast (beef), skinless thighs (chicken)	

FISH COUNTER	GRAINS
Aim for two servings per person per week Filet: Allow 4 ounces per portion Whole fish: Allow 8 ounces per portion (Portion = 3 ounces cooked fish) **Best Choices** **Fresh:** arctic char, wild salmon, sablefish (black cod), oysters (farmed) **Frozen:** wild salmon, shrimp **Canned:** wild Alaska pink salmon, Alaskan sockeye, sardines, anchovies **Budget –friendly:** cod, haddock, chunk light tuna	**Higher in protein:** teff, amaranth, quinoa **Higher in fiber:** bulgur, brown rice **Lower in carbohydrates and calories:** buckwheat, bulgur, polenta, oats, wild rice **Lower glycemic load :** basmati rice **Higher in calcium and iron:** amaranth, teff **Higher in omega-3:** quinoa, wild rice

PASTA	FLOUR
Higher in protein: "Plus" brand (with legume flour), egg noodles **Higher in fiber:** whole wheat **Lower in carbohydrates:** egg, whole wheat **Lower in calories:** quinoa	White whole wheat flour offers all the nutritional advantages of whole grain flour but is lighter in flavor and texture than regular whole wheat flour. When modifying recipes, white whole wheat flour makes a better substitute for white flour than regular whole wheat flour does.

BREADS	CEREAL
Look for whole grain breads that contain at least 3 grams of fiber per serving.	Look for cereal with less than 5 grams of sugar and 5 grams or more of fiber per serving.

SWEETENERS	SPICES AND SEASONINGS
Sugar **Least refined:** raw sugar **Best substitute for white sugar:** evaporated cane juice **Most eco-friendly:** organic **Liquid Sugar** **Most nutrients**: molasses **Lowest in calories:** maple syrup **Least effect on blood sugar:** agave, honey	Unrefined (gourmet) salts contain trace minerals and can be lower in sodium than refined salt. When sprinkling salt on top of a finished dish, kosher salt gives you more flavor with less sodium. If you prefer not to use iodized salt, be sure there are other sources of iodine in your diet.

SWEETENERS	SPICES AND SEASONINGS
Artificial Sweeteners **Most satural/safest:** stevia, erythritol **Best (but not ideal) for baking:** erythritol, sucralose (Splenda) **Least aftertaste:** erythritol, sucralose (Splenda)	Potassium chloride is a safe and natural option for those who need to avoid all sodium. It tastes salty, but can have a bitter or metallic aftertaste. **Super Spices:** **Antioxidant activity:** clove, allspice **Blood sugar control:** cinnamon **Anti-inflammatory activity:** curry powder, turmeric, ginger, garlic **Appetite regulation:** red pepper flakes, cayenne pepper
OILS	VINEGAR
Best for overall nutrition: extra-virgin olive oil **Best for neutral flavor:** canola (expeller-pressed) **Best for gourmet touches:** hazelnut, walnut **Best for high-heat cooking:** palm kernel, high-heat canola	If you're trying to keep it simple, cider and balsamic vinegar will cover most of your needs. Salad dressings made with milder vinegars like balsamic and rice vinegar require less oil. Herb and fruit vinegars add flavor and interest to sauces and salad dressings.
SALAD DRESSING	MAYONNAISE
Choose vinaigrette-style dressings made with recognizable ingredients. Avoid thick, creamy salad dressings and those with lots of artificial additives.	Mayonnaise made with canola or olive oil is a better choice than mayonnaise made with soybean oil. If calories are a concern, choose light (not fat-free) mayo and look for the brand with the fewest artificial ingredients.
NUTS, SEEDS, AND NUT BUTTERS	DRIED BEANS
Higher in protein: peanuts, pumpkin seeds **Higher in fiber:** chia, flax, almonds **Higher in phytosterols (cholesterol-lowering compounds):** sesame, sunflower, pistachio **Higher in omega-3s:** flax, chia, walnuts **Higher in calcium:** sesame, chia, almonds **Lower in fat and calories:** chestnuts, pumpkin, cashews Look for butters made with ground nuts or seeds and not much else.	**Higher in protein:** white (by a small amount) **Higher in fiber:** navy, pinto, black, cranberry **Lower in calories and carbohydrates:** fava, lentil, split pea **Higher in iron:** white, lentil, garbanzo, **Higher in folic acid:** cranberry, lentil, garbanzo, pinto

DRIED FRUIT	CANNED VEGETABLES
High in antioxidants: blueberries, cherries, apricots **Higher in fiber:** persimmons, apples, figs **Lower in sugar:** apricots, prunes, figs **Higher in iron:** apricots, prunes	To reduce BPA exposure, use fresh or frozen vegetables and dried beans rather than canned vegetables and beans whenever possible. Buy tomatoes in glass jars or aseptic packaging.

Serving Size Guide

VEGETABLES (25–75 CALORIES)
8 large lettuce leaves
1 cup (packed) baby spinach or other greens (about the size of a baseball)
½ cup cooked vegetables (size of an ice-cream scoop)
1 bell pepper or tomato
½ large cucumber or zucchini
1 large handful cut-up raw vegetables
½ cup coleslaw or broccoli salad (size of an ice-cream scoop)
bowl of vegetable soup

FRUITS (50 TO 100 CALORIES)
1 cup berries, grapes, or cut up fruit
1 apple, peach, orange, or banana
2 apricots or plums
½ cup fruit juice
¼ to ⅓ cup dried fruit

FATS AND OILS (80–120 CALORIES)
1 tablespoon regular mayonnaise or salad dressing
¼ avocado
2 tablespoons light mayo or dressing
2 tablespoons sour cream
1 tablespoon butter or oil

GRAINS/STARCHES (80–120 CALORIES)
1 slice bread
1 small pita
1 medium flour tortilla
1 small roll
4-6 crackers
⅓ cup potato or pasta salad (about the size of a large egg)

PROTEIN FOODS (150–200 CALORIES)
3 ounces sliced turkey or roast beef (3 medium-thick slices)
3 ounces cooked fish, poultry, or meat (about the size of a deck of cards)
2 hard-boiled eggs
1 small (3 to 4 ounce) can tuna, sardines, salmon
½ cup tuna, chicken, egg, or tofu salad (size of an ice-cream scoop)
1 ounce hard cheese (size of your thumb or a CD without the case)
½ cup cottage cheese or yogurt (size of an ice-cream scoop)
2 tablespoons nut butter (about the size of a golf ball)
bowl of bean or split pea soup

Guide to Cooking Methods

COOKING METHOD	DESCRIPTION	USE FOR	GOOD PICK?
Steam	Cooked over boiling water	vegetables	Preserves nutrients and texture in vegetables
Boil/ blanch	Cooked in boiling water	vegetables pasta eggs	Adds no fat Cook vegetables only until tender to preserve nutrients
Poach	Cooked gently in water or a thin liquid (such as milk or wine)	eggs fish fruit	Adds little or no fat Good for delicate foods
Bake	Cooked in a dry, medium heat	meat fish casseroles potatoes baked goods	Hands-off method is convenient Sauces, coatings, and toppings may add fat and/or calories
Braise	Cooked slowly in liquid such as wine or stock	meats vegetables	Good for tenderizing tougher vegetables or cuts of meat
Roast	Cooked with dry, medium-high heat	meat poultry vegetables	Concentrates flavor in vegetables Reduces fat in meat and poultry
Broil/grill	Cooked with direct, high heat	meat fish vegetables	Adds flavor Sauces may add fat and calories Marinate meats and avoid flare ups and excessive charring
Sautée	Cooked in small amount of oil or butter over medium heat	vegetables smaller pieces of meat	Quick cooking method is convenient and preserves nutrients in vegetables Avoid excessive amounts of oil
Stir-fry	Cooked in small amount of oil over high heat	vegetables smaller pieces of meat	Quick cooking method preserves nutrients and texture in vegetables Avoid excessive amounts of oil
Deep-fry	Cooked in large amount of oil at high temperature	fish potatoes battered vegetables	High in fat and calories May contain significant amount of trans fats Best avoided

ACKNOWLEDGMENTS

MY THANKS TO all the people who helped make this book possible: my skilled and gracious editor, Emily Rothschild, and her assistant, Greg Baird; Kim Baker and Christy Paulley, who tested several of the recipes; Mignon "Grammar Girl" Fogarty, whose entrepreneurial talents launched the Quick and Dirty Tips network; Richard Rhorer, to whom we owe the ongoing success and growth of the QDT project; our podcast sponsors; my fellow Quick and Dirty Tips hosts, for their help and inspiration; to my sweetheart, family, and friends, for their patience and support, especially during that final six weeks of writing—which is never pretty; and to all of the listeners, readers, Facebook fans, and Twitter followers, whose ideas, opinions, questions, and suggestions shaped this book. Read it in good health (and please buy copies for all your friends!).

INDEX

acesulfame k, 66
acetic acid, 77, 79
acid-forming foods, 195–196
additives
  butter sprays, 30
  dairy products, 20, 25
  grains, 49
  low-carb bars, 155
  margarine, 28
  mayonnaise, 77
  microwave popcorn, 97
  nuts and seeds, 81
  salad dressings, 80
agar, 20
agave syrup, 63, 64
agricultural chemicals, 9–11,
  58, 73, 75
albacore tuna, 40, 41
alcoholic beverages, 174–176
allergens, 21, 22, 82
all-purpose white flour, 58
allspice, 70, 218
almond butter, 81–82
almond milk, 21
almond oil, 71
almonds, 81
alphalinoleic acid (ALA), 188
Alzheimer's disease, 193
amaranth, 49, 50, 60
American Heart Association
  (AHA), 178, 192–193
amino acids, 30, 66, 160
anchovies, 40, 43
antibiotics, 17, 31, 35, 36–37
anti-inflammatory activity, 70
antinutrients, 24
antioxidants
  dried fruit, 82, 83
  herbs, 12, 70
  oils, 71
  produce, 7
appetite control, 52, 70
apples
  Apple Pie Oatmeal, 198
  dried fruit, 83
  fruit juice, 32

pesticide residues, 10
seasonality, 9
shelf-life, 13
shopping tips, 13
snacks, 150–151
apricots, 8, 9, 83, 150–151
Arctic char, 43
artichokes, 9, 84
artificial sweeteners
  benefits, 64–65
  best choices, 67
  diet drinks, 103–104
  low-carb bars, 155
  safety concerns, 65
  varieties, 66–67
  weight management issues,
  65–66
arugula, 8
aseptic packaging, 84, 85
Asian-style Broccoli Salad, 204
asparagus, 9, 209
aspartame, 66
avocado oil, 71

babies, nutritional concerns, 23,
  38, 41, 84
baby greens, 9
bacon, 37, 38, 120–121
bacteria, 24–25
bakeries, 128
balsamic vinegar, 78, 79
bananas, 13, 52, 122, 124, 150
barley, 49, 53
basil, 12
basmati rice, 48
beans, 9, 13, 219, 220
  See also dried beans
beef
  Chili Con Cocoo, 220
  hormones, 37–38
  Moroccan Sliders, 217
  red versus white meat,
  33, 34
  shopping tips, 228
beer, 175, 176
beet greens, 7

beets, 9
bell peppers, 7, 8, 10
beneficial bacteria, 24–25
berries, 7, 9, 10, 13, 122, 124
Best Fruit and Nut Bars, 206
beta carotene, 150, 182
beverages
  alcoholic beverages, 174–176
  bottled water, 98–100
  caffeinated beverages,
  107–112
  diet drinks, 103–104
  fruit and vitamin waters, 104
  mineral water, 100
  soda, 102–103
  sports drinks, 190
  water, 98
  water filters, 101
bigeye tuna, 42
bioengineering, 73
bison, 34, 217, 220, 228
bisphenol A (BPA), 84–85
black beans, 83
black cod, 40, 43
blood sugar regulation, 53, 70,
  144–145, 167
blood type diet, 193–194
blueberries, 83, 122
blue cheese, 27
bluefin tuna, 40, 42
bluefish, 42
bologna, 38
bottled salad dressings, 80
bottled water, 98–100
bowel function, 52
Braised Fennel, 212
bran, 46, 58
bread flour, 59
breads, 54–56, 127, 132–133, 229
breakfast, 107–128, 223–226
Breakfast Burrito, 201
breakfast cereals, 56–58
break times, 136
breast cancer, 15, 22–23
broccoli, 7, 8, 9, 13, 14, 204
brown rice, 48

brown rice syrup, 63, 64
brown sugar, 61
brussels sprouts, 7, 8, 9
buckwheat, 49, 50, 60
bulgur, 49, 50
burgers, 138, 139
Burrito, Breakfast, 201
butter, 28–30, 76, 127, 228
buttermilk, 24
butters, nut and seed, 81–82,
    127, 230
butter sprays, 30

cabbage, 7, 8, 9
caffeine, 107–112
cage-free eggs and poultry, 31,
    34–35
calcium
    cheese, 27
    cooking method effects, 162
    cultured dairy products, 24
    daily requirements, 184–185
    dairy products, 14, 15
    fish, 14
    grains, 49–50
    Greek-style yogurt, 26
    kale, 7
    molasses, 64
    nondairy milk products, 22
    nuts and seeds, 81
    produce, 14
    soda, 103
calories
    alcoholic beverages, 175, 176
    breakfast recommendations,
        125–127
    butter sprays, 30
    cheese, 26–27
    chocolate, 180
    dairy products, 18, 19,
        126–127
    desserts, 177
    dinner recommendations,
        169
    dried beans, 83
    eggs, 126
    fat-burning exercise,
        112–113
    grains, 49–50, 165
    Greek-style yogurt, 26
    liquid sweeteners, 63–64
    mayonnaise, 77
    nondairy milk products, 21
    nut and seed butters, 81–82,
        127
    Nutrition Facts label, 91–92
    nuts and seeds, 81, 127,
        152–153
    post-exercise meals, 190–191

reduced-fat dairy spreads, 29
resistant starches, 53
smoothies, 124
snacks, 147–148, 153, 172–173
soda, 103
vinegars, 77
Camembert cheese, 27
Canadian bacon, 127
cancer
    artificial sweeteners, 65
    dairy products, 15
    diet trends, 193
    nitrates/nitrites, 38
    polychlorinated biphenyls
        (PCBs), 41
    refined grains, 46
    soymilk, 22–23
canned fish, 43, 44
canned vegetables, 84–85, 231
cannellini beans, 83
canola oil, 71, 72–73, 75–76, 77
cantaloupe, 8, 9
carbohydrates
    breakfast choices, 115–116
    cooking tips, 165–169
    daily servings, 232
    Daily Values (DVs), 92
    energy bars, 153–156
    food-combination myths,
        133–134
    low-carb diets, 191–192, 193
    post-exercise meals, 190–191
    See also grains; produce;
        sugar
carbonated water, 99
carotenoids, 150
carrots, 7, 8, 9, 13, 149
carry-out
    See takeout
cashew butter, 81–82
cashews, 81
cauliflower, 7, 8, 9, 149, 210,
    211
caviar, 40
cayenne pepper, 70, 218, 219
celery, 10, 149
celiac disease, 53–54
cereals, 56–58, 229
chain restaurants, 139–140
chard, 7, 8, 9, 215
cheese, 26–28, 127, 152, 200,
    228
    See also dairy products
cherries, 8, 10, 83
chestnuts, 81
chia seeds, 74, 81, 188
chicken, 33, 38, 216, 228
Chicken, Crunchy Sesame
    Flax, 216

children, nutritional concerns,
    10, 38, 41, 84
Chilean sea bass, 42
Chili Con Cocoa, 220
chili powder, 220
Chinese food, 136–137, 138
chips, 95–96
chocolate, 179–180
cholesterol, 32, 77, 117, 119
cider vinegar, 78, 79
cinnamon, 70, 218
citrus, 8, 9, 13, 32, 33
clementines, 9
cloves, 70, 218
club soda, 99
cobie, 42
cocoa powder, 123, 124, 220
coconut oil, 71, 75–76
cod, 43
coffee, 107–112, 122–123
coffee-flavored yogurt, 25
coffee shops, 128
cold cuts, 38
cold-pressed oils, 75
collards, 8
conventional versus organic
        products
    dairy products, 16–17
    eggs, 31
    meat, 35
    produce, 11–12
converted rice, 48
cookies, 95–96
cooking liquid, 163
cooking method guide, 233
coriander, 218
corn, 7, 9, 84
corn oil, 74
cottage cheese, 27, 126
couscous, 51
crackers, 95–96
Cranberries, Quinoa Salad with
        Pecans and, 214
cranberry beans, 83
cream cheese, 228
cream, fat-free, 20
creamy salad dressings, 80
croaker, 42
Crunchy Sesame Flax Chicken,
    216
cucumbers, 9, 149
cultured dairy products, 24–26
cumin, 218, 219
cured meats, 38
curry powder
    Curried Tuna Salad, 205
    health benefits, 70
    Sweet Potato and
        Cauliflower Curry, 210

Daily Values (DVs), 92–93
dairy cows, 37–38
dairy products
    butter, 28–30
    cheese, 26–28
    daily servings, 27
    fat-free cream, 20
    health benefits, 15–16
    lactose-free milk, 19
    nutritional value, 14,
        126–127
    organic products, 16–17
    reduced-fat dairy products,
        18–19, 20
    shelf-life, 27
    shopping tips, 27–28, 228
    snacks, 152
    unnatural consumption, 16
    yogurt, 24–26
    See also nondairy milk
        products
deli meats, 38, 228
deli shops, 137–138, 139
demerara sugar, 61
depression, 193
desserts, 95, 176–180
diabetes
    artificial sweeteners, 67
    blood sugar regulation, 145
    diet trends, 193
    refined grains, 46
    resistant starches, 53
diet drinks, 103–104
diet makeover
    See 24-hour diet makeover
diet trends, 191–196
digestive system, 133–134, 151
diners, 127–128
dinner, 157–173, 223–226
Dirty Dozen, 10
distilled vinegar, 78
distilled water, 99
dried beans, 52, 83, 158, 230
dried fruit, 82–83, 150–151,
    206, 231

eating frequency, 146–147
eggplant, 9
eggs
    cholesterol, 32, 119
    cooking methods, 233
    Leftover Vegetable Frittata,
        200
    mayonnaise, 77
    microwave cooking, 120
    nutritional value, 30–32, 126
    shopping tips, 228
endive, 9
endosperm, 46

energy bars, 153–156, 190
enhanced milk, 19
Environmental Defense Fund
    (EDF), 42
Environmental Working
    Group, 10
Equal, 66
erucic acid, 72
erythritol, 66–67
esterified oils, 28, 29
esters, 28, 29
estrogen-sensitive tumors, 23
evaporated cane juice, 61, 62
exercise, 112–113, 147, 178,
    189–191
expeller pressed oils, 75
extra-virgin olive oil, 71, 76

farmed fish, 42
fast food, 128, 138, 139
fat
    See oils
fat-burning exercise, 112–113
fat-free cream, 20
fava beans, 83
fed state, 146
fennel, 14, 212
Fennel, Braised, 212
fermented soy products, 24
feta cheese, 27, 28
fetuses, nutritional concerns,
    38, 41, 110
fiber
    breads, 55–56
    breakfast recommendations,
        117, 125–127
    cereals, 58
    Daily Values (DVs), 93
    dairy products, 126–127
    dietary recommendations,
        117
    dried beans, 83
    dried fruit, 83
    eggs, 126
    energy bars, 153–156
    flaxseeds, 123, 124
    fruit juice, 32
    grains, 49
    nondairy milk products, 21
    nuts and seeds, 81, 127
    oatmeal, 57
    pasta, 51
    red bell peppers, 6
    resistant starches, 52
    smoothies, 123, 124
    soluble versus insoluble
        fiber, 116–117
figs, 83, 150, 208
filtered oils, 75

filtered water, 98–99
filters, water, 101
fish
    best choices, 43
    breakfast choices, 125
    cooking methods, 233
    Curried Tuna Salad, 205
    daily servings, 40, 44
    Fish Soup, 221
    frozen and canned fish,
        43, 44
    health benefits, 40, 74
    mercury levels, 40–41
    nutritional value, 14
    polychlorinated biphenyls
        (PCBs), 41–42
    seafood guides, 42–43
    shelf-life and storage, 44
    shopping tips, 44, 229
    sustainability, 42
fish oil supplements, 186–187
flavanols, 123, 179–180
flax, 74, 81
flaxseed oil, 71
flaxseeds, 123, 124, 188, 206,
    216
flounder, 42
flour, 50–51, 58–60, 229
folate, 6, 162
folic acid, 50, 83, 182–183
food-combination myths,
    133–134
free-range eggs and poultry,
    31, 34–35
Frittata, Leftover Vegetable, 201
frozen fish, 43, 44
frozen foods, 135–136
frozen fruits and vegetables,
    12–13, 84, 85, 122
frozen meat, 39
frozen yogurt, 25
fructose, 64
fruits/fruit juice
    best choices, 7–8
    Best Fruit and Nut Bars, 206
    cooking methods, 233
    costs, 6, 8
    daily servings, 13, 232
    dried fruit, 82–83, 150–151,
        206, 231
    fortified water, 104
    frozen fruits, 12–13, 122
    Goat Cheese Spread with Figs
        and Black Pepper, 208
    nutritional value, 32–33, 127,
        150–151
    organic produce, 9–11
    Quinoa Salad with Pecans
        and Cranberries, 214

fruits/fruit juice (continued)
    seasonality, 8–9
    serving quantity, 5–6
    shelf-life, 13
    shopping tips, 13–14, 227,
        228
    smoothies, 121, 122
    snacks, 150–152
    sugar content, 90
    washing, 11
fruit vinegars, 79

garbanzo beans, 83
garlic, 7, 8, 9, 70
gastrointestinal distress, 52
genetically modified organisms
    (GMOs), 73
germ, 46, 58
ginger, 70, 218
glass packaging, 84, 85
gluten flour, 59
gluten-free products
    benefits, 53–54
    flour, 60
    grains, 49
    pasta, 51
glycemic load, 46, 48, 51, 57,
    167
goat cheese, 27, 208
Goat Cheese Spread with
    Figs and Black Pepper,
    208
Gouda cheese, 27
gourmet salt, 69
grains
    benefits, 45–46
    best choices, 50
    breads, 54–56
    cooking tips, 165–169
    daily servings, 47, 165–166,
        232
    gluten-free products, 49,
        53–54
    intact versus milled grains,
        46–47
    rice, 47–48
    shopping tips, 229
    whole-grain foods, 46–47
granola, 116
grapefruit, 9
grapes, 7, 8, 10, 32, 33
grapeseed oil, 71
grass-fed/grass-finished beef,
    34, 36
Greek-style yogurt, 26
green beans, 7, 13
greens, 7, 8, 9, 13, 14
green tea, 111–112, 122–123
grilling tips, 160–161

grocery shopping
    challenges, 3
    packaged and prepared
        foods, 86–104
    pantry staples, 45–85
    perimeter shopping, 5–44
grouper, 42
Gruyère cheese, 27
Guacamole, Tomatillo, 207
guar gum, 20

haddock, 43
ham, 38, 120–121
hard sausages, 38
hazelnut oil, 71, 76
health halo effect, 96
healthy food selection, 1–2
heart disease, 23, 46, 110, 193
hemp milk, 21
hemp seeds, 74, 188
herbal vinegars, 79
herbicides
    flour, 58
    genetically engineered
        foods, 73
    oils, 75
    produce, 9–11
    sugar, 62
herbs, 8, 12, 13, 70
herring, 40
heterocyclic amines (HCAs),
    160, 161
high-fructose corn syrup, 90–91
high-smoke point oils, 75–76
hi-maize flour, 60
honey, 63, 64, 90, 123, 124
hormones, 16–17, 35, 37–38
hot cereals, 57
hot dogs, 38
humanely-raised meats, 35
hunger symptoms, 115,
    146–147
hydrogenated oils, 28, 29, 76, 89

imitation butter sprays, 30
Indian food, 137, 139, 170
ingredient liss, 87–88
injected meats, 33
insoluble fiber, 116–117
instant oatmeal, 57
instant rice, 48
intact versus milled grains,
    46–47
interesterified fats, 28, 29
iodized salt, 68
iron, 33, 49–50, 64, 83
isoflavones, 22
Israeli couscous, 51
Italian food, 138, 139

Japanese food, 137, 139, 170
jasmine rice, 48
juices, 32–33

kale, 7, 8, 9, 13, 213
kamut flour, 59
kasha, 49
kefir, 24–26
king mackerel, 41
kiwi, 8
Kosher meats, 35
Kosher salt, 69

lactose-free milk, 19
lamb, 34, 228
late-night snacks, 172–173
leafy greens, 7, 8, 14
leeks, 9
Leftover Vegetable Frittata, 200
legumes, 51, 53, 82
lemon-flavored yogurt, 25
lemons, 9
lentils, 51, 83
lettuce, 7, 9, 10, 13
limes, 9
liquid sweeteners, 63–64
liquor, 175, 176
live and active cultured dairy
    products, 24–25
livestock
    See meat
long-grain rice, 48
Louisiana Red Beans and
    Rice, 219
low-caloric breads, 56
low-carb bars, 155
low-carb diets, 191–192, 193
low-fat dairy products, 18–19,
    20, 25
low-sodium salt alternatives, 69
lunch, 129–141, 223–226
lycopene, 13, 150

mackerel, 40, 41
magnesium, 15
maltitol, 66
malt vinegar, 78
mangos, 52, 122
maple syrup, 64, 123, 124
margarine, 28, 228
marlin, 42
mayonnaise, 77, 230
meal plans, 105–106, 223–226
meal replacement bars, 154–155
meals on the fly, 14, 39, 44
meat
    antibiotics use, 35, 36–37
    best choices, 34
    breakfast choices, 120–121

Chili Con Cocoa, 220
cold cuts/cured meats, 38
cooking tips, 160–161, 233
    daily servings, 39
    frozen meat, 39
    hormones, 35, 37–38
    labeling guide, 34–35
    Moroccan Sliders, 217
    portion size, 39
    red versus white meat, 33
    shopping tips, 39, 228–229
    See also poultry
Mediterranean diet, 192–193
melons, 8, 9, 13
men and soy products, 23
menu decoder, 170
mercury, 40–41
mesclun mix, 9
metabolism, 130, 143–144, 146
Mexican food, 137, 138–139
microwave cooking, 120,
    135, 163
microwave popcorn, 97
milk, 18–19, 122, 124, 126, 228
    See also dairy products
milled grains, 46–47
millet, 49, 60
minerals
    bottled water, 98–100
    cooking method effects,
        162–163
    dairy products, 15
    dried beans/dried fruit, 83
    health benefits, 183
    meat, 33
    molasses, 64
    oatmeal, 57
mineral water, 100
miso, 24
mixed drinks, 175, 176
molasses, 64, 90
monkfish, 42
monounsaturated fats, 33, 71
Monsanto, 73
Monterey Bay Aquarium, 43
Monterey jack cheese, 28
Moroccan Sliders, 217
mozzarella cheese, 27, 28
muesli, 116
multigrain porridge, 57
multivitamins, 181–184
mushrooms, 7, 8
mustard greens, 7
mystery water, 99

natto, 24
naturally occurring trans fats, 89
natural versus refined sugar,
    60–61

navy beans, 83
nectarines, 9, 10
nitrates/nitrites, 38, 120–121
noncarbonated soft drinks,
    103–104
nondairy milk products, 20–24,
    228
nonwheat flours, 59–60
nut oils, 74
Nutrasweet, 66
nutritional supplements,
    181–189, 191
Nutritional Yeast, Tofu Salad
    with, 203
Nutrition Facts label, 91–93, 94,
    96, 177–178
nuts and seeds
    Best Fruit and Nut Bars, 206
    fruit pairings, 151–152
    nutritional value, 80–82, 127
    omega-6 fatty acids, 187
    Quinoa Salad with Pecans
        and Cranberries, 214
    shopping tips, 230
    snacks, 152–153

oatmeal, 57, 118, 126, 127,
    198–199
oat milk, 21
oats, 49, 50, 60, 198–199
obesity, 46, 90–91, 103
oils
    best choices, 76
    cooking needs, 74
    daily servings, 232
    fat varieties, 71
    genetically engineered foods,
        72–73
    health benefits, 74
    high-heat cooking, 75–76
    hydrogenated oils, 28, 29,
        76, 89
    labeling guide, 74–75
    mayonnaise, 77
    partially hydrogenated
        vegetable oil, 76, 88–89
    shopping tips, 230
    shortening, 76
olive oil, 71, 75, 76, 77
olives, 84
omega-3 fatty acids
    beef, 34
    canola oil, 72
    eggs, 30–31
    fish, 40, 186–187
    health benefits, 74, 186–188
    hemp milk, 21
    margarine, 28–29
    nuts and seeds, 81, 188

pastured meats, 35
    wild rice, 50
omega-6 fatty acids, 74, 77, 187
onions, 7, 8, 9
orange roughy, 42
oranges, 9, 13
oregano, 12
organic cane sugar, 62
organic dairy products, 16–17
organic eggs, 31
organic flour, 58
organic meats, 35
organic oils, 75
organic produce, 9–12
organic shortening, 76
osteoporosis, 15–16
oxalates, 24, 123
oysters, 43

packaged and prepared foods
    beverages, 98–104
    hydrogenated oils, 89
    ingredients, 87–88
    Nutrition Facts label, 91–93,
        94, 96
    shopping tips, 86
    sweet and salty treats, 95–97
    sweeteners, 90–91, 177–179
    takeout, 93–95, 136–139
    trans fats, 88–89
palm kernel oil, 71, 75–76
pancake houses, 127–128
pantry staples
    breads, 54–56
    canned vegetables, 84–85
    cereals, 56–58
    dried beans, 83
    dried fruit, 82–83
    flour, 58–60
    grains, 45–50
    herbs and spices, 70
    oils, 71–77
    pasta, 50–54
    salt, 68–70
    shelf-life, 85
    shopping tips, 85
    sweeteners, 60–67
    vinegars, 77–80
Parkinson's disease, 193
Parmesan cheese, 27
parsley, 12
parsnips, 9
partially hydrogenated
    vegetable oil, 76, 88–89
part-skim ricotta cheese, 27
pasta
    blood sugar regulation,
        167–168
    cooking methods, 233

pasta *(continued)*
  nutritional value, 50–52
  Penne with Sautéed Chard, 215
  portion size, 167
  Salmon and Rotini Salad, 202
  shopping tips, 229
pastry flour, whole-wheat, 59
pastured eggs, 31
pastured meats, 35, 36
PCBs
  See polychlorinated biphenyls (PCBs)
peaches, 9, 10, 13, 122, 124
peanut butter, 81–82, 122, 124, 206
peanut oil, 74
peanuts, 81, 82
pears, 9, 10
peas, 7, 9, 51
Pecans and Cranberries, Quinoa Salad with, 214
Penne with Sautéed Chard, 215
perimeter shopping
  dairy products, 14–20, 24–30
  eggs, 30–32
  fish, 40–44
  meat, 33–39
  nondairy milk products, 20–24
  produce, 5–14
persimmons, 83
pesticides
  dairy products, 16
  eggs, 31
  flour, 58
  meat, 35
  oils, 75
  produce, 9–11
  sugar, 62
pH-balancing diet, 195–196
phosphates, 15, 103
phytates, 24
phytochemicals, 12
phytoestrogens, 22–23
phytosterols, 28–29, 81
pilaf cooking method, 167
pinto beans, 83
pistachios, 81
pizzas, 138, 139
plain yogurt, 25
plant sterols, 80, 152
polenta, 50
polychlorinated biphenyls (PCBs), 41–42
polycyclic aromatic hydrocarbons (PAHs), 160
polyphenols, 71, 175

polyunsaturated fats, 71, 74
  See also omega-3 fatty acids
pomegranates, 8, 9, 32, 33
popcorn, 97
pork, 33, 34, 37, 228
postabsorptive state, 146
post-exercise meals, 190–191
potassium chloride, 69
potatoes, 7, 9, 10, 52, 233
poultry
  best choices, 34
  cooking methods, 233
  Crunchy Sesame Flax Chicken, 216
  hormones, 37
  red versus white meat, 33
  shopping tips, 228
prebasted meats, 33
pregnant women, nutritional concerns, 38, 41, 84, 110
pretzels, 95
processed foods
  hydrogenated oils, 89
  ingredients, 87–88
  nut and seed butters, 81–82, 127
  salt content, 70
  shopping tips, 86
  sweeteners, 90–91
  trans fats, 88–89
processed fruit juice, 32–33
produce
  best choices, 7–8
  cooking methods, 233
  costs, 6, 8
  daily servings, 13, 232
  frozen fruits and vegetables, 12–13
  herbs, 8, 12
  organic produce, 9–11
  seasonality, 8–9
  serving quantity, 5–6
  shelf-life, 13
  shopping tips, 13–14, 227
  washing, 11
prostate cancer, 23
protein
  breakfast recommendations, 118–121, 125–127
  cheese, 27
  cultured dairy products, 24
  daily requirements, 118–119, 131–132, 232
  Daily Values (DVs), 92–93
  dairy products, 14, 126–127
  dinner, 158
  dried beans, 83
  eggs, 30, 31, 32, 126
  energy bars, 153–156

fish, 14
flour, 59
food-combination myths, 133–134
grains, 49–50, 165
Greek-style yogurt, 26
lunch recommendations, 130
meat, 33
metabolic effects, 130
nondairy milk products, 20–21
nuts and seeds, 80–81, 127
pasta, 51
post-exercise meals, 190–191
smoothies, 122, 124
prunes, 83, 150–151
pumpkins, 9
pumpkin seeds, 81
Purevia, 67

quinoa, 50, 51, 214
Quinoa Salad with Pecans and Cranberries, 214

radicchio, 9
radishes, 9, 13, 149
rainbow trout, 40, 42
raisins, 150
rancid oils, 74
rapeseed oil, 72
Ras El Hanout, 218
raspberries, 122
raw foods, 13, 164–165
raw sugar, 60–61, 62
rBST, 16
ready-to-eat cereals, 56–57
recovery meals, 190–191
red beans, 83, 219
red bell peppers, 6, 7, 8, 149
red meat
  See meat
red pepper flakes, 70
reduced-fat dairy products, 18–19, 20
reduced-fat dairy spreads, 29
reduced-fat mayonnaise, 77
reduced-fat nut butters, 81–82
red wine, 175, 176
refined grains, 46–47, 54
refined oils, 75
refined white sugar, 60–61
regularity, 52
resistant starches, 52–53, 60
restaurant meals, 136–141, 169–172
resveratrol, 7
rhubarb, 9
rice, 47–48, 51, 52, 60, 219
rice milk, 21, 126

rice vinegar/rice wine vinegar, 78
ricotta cheese, 27
roast beef, 38
Roasted Cauliflower, 211
rockfish, 42
rosemary, 12
Roundup, 73
Rule of Five, 57
rutabagas, 9
rye, 53

sablefish, 40, 43
saccharine, 67
safflower oil, 74
salad bars, 140–141
salad dressing, 80, 230
  See also vinegars
salads
  Asian-style Broccoli Salad, 204
  Curried Tuna Salad, 205
  Quinoa Salad with Pecans and Cranberries, 214
  Salmon and Rotini Salad, 202
  Tofu Salad with Nutritional Yeast, 203
salami, 38
salmon, 14, 40, 43, 127, 202
Salmon and Rotini Salad, 202
salt
  Daily Values (DVs), 93
  deli meats, 38
  nondairy milk products, 22
  nut and seed butters, 81–82
  processed foods, 70
  sweet and salty treats, 95–97
  varieties, 68 69
sample meal plans, 223–226
sandwich shops, 137–138, 139
sardines, 14, 40, 43
saturated fats, 18–19, 28, 71
sausage, 120–121, 127
Sautéed Chard, Penne with, 215
scallions, 7, 9
scrambled eggs, 120
seafood
  See fish
seafood guides, 42–43
sea salt, 68
seasoned rice vinegar, 79
seaweed, 20
seed oils, 74
seeds
  See nuts and seeds
selective breeding programs, 72–73
selenium, 183–184

seltzer water, 99, 100
serving size guide, 232
sesame oil, 71, 74
sesame seeds, 81, 216
shallots, 7
shark, 41, 42
shellfish, 40
shopping guide, 227–231
shortening, 76
short-grain rice, 48
shrimp, 43
Silken Asparagus Soup, 209
skim milk, 18–19
smoothies, 121–124, 126
snacks
  calorie budget, 147–148
  dairy products, 27–28
  eating frequency, 146 147
  food choices, 148–156
  late-night snacks, 172–173
  meal plans, 223–226
  nuts and seeds, 80
  prevalence, 142–143
  produce, 13
  sweet and salty treats, 95–97
snow peas, 7, 13, 149
soda, 102–103
sodium
  cheese, 27
  Daily Values (DVs), 93
  dairy products, 15
  deli meats, 38
  grains, 49
  nondairy milk products, 22
  processed foods, 70
  sweet and salty treats, 95–97
  See also salt
soluble fiber, 116–117
sorbitol, 66–67
soup, 209, 221
sour cream, 228
sourdough breads, 55
soybean oil, 71, 74, 77
soybeans, 24
soymilk, 20–21, 122, 124, 126
soy-nut butter, 82
soy sauce, 24
spaghetti squash, 168
specialty oils, 74
spelt flour, 59
spices, 70, 217, 218, 229–230
spinach, 7, 10, 24, 123, 124
Splenda, 67
split peas, 83
sport nutrition bars, 154
sports drinks, 190
spray butters, 30
spreadable butter, 29
spring water, 99

sprouted-grain breads, 55
squash, 7, 8, 9, 13
standard couscous, 51
starch
  See carbohydrates
starvation mode, 143
steamed grains, 166
steamed vegetables, 163
steel-cut oats, 49, 57
stevia, 67, 123
strawberries, 10, 122, 124
striped bass, 42
sturgeon, 42
sucralose, 67
sugar
  best choices, 62
  cereals, 57, 58
  Daily Values (DVs), 93
  desserts, 176–180
  dietary consumption, 62–63
  dietary recommendations, 177–179
  dried fruit, 83
  fruit and vitamin waters, 104
  fruit juice, 32–33
  nondairy milk products, 21, 22
  nut and seed butters, 81–82
  nutritional value, 60–61
  packaged and prepared foods, 90–91, 177–179
  soda, 102–103
  sugar substitutes, 64–67
  sweet and salty treats, 95–97
  varieties, 61–62
sugar alcohols, 66–67
sugar snap peas, 149
sulfites, 82
summer squash, 9
sunflower oil, 74
sunflower seed butter, 81–82
sunflower seeds, 81
Sunnett, 66
sushi, 137, 139, 170
sustainable fishing practices, 42
sweetened yogurt, 25
sweeteners
  artificial sweeteners, 64–67
  best choices, 62, 64
  diet drinks, 103–104
  fruit and vitamin waters, 104
  liquid sweeteners, 63–64
  packaged and prepared foods, 90–91, 177–179
  shopping tips, 229–230
  smoothies, 123
  soda, 102–103
  sugar, 60–63
  sweet and salty treats, 95–97

Sweet'N Low, 67
Sweet One, 66
Sweet Potato and Cauliflower
    Curry, 210
sweet potatoes, 7, 8, 210
Swerve, 66
Swiss chard, 7, 8, 9
Swiss cheese, 27
swordfish, 41, 42
synthetic fertilizers, 9–10
synthetic sweeteners, 66–67
syrups, 90

table salt, 68
takeout, 93–95, 136–139
tangerines, 9
tap water, 98
tea, 107–112
teff, 50
tempeh, 24
Tender Kale, 213
testosterone, 23
thermic effect of food, 143–144
thyroid function, 23
tilefish, 41, 42
toasted oils, 75
tofu, 122, 124, 127, 203, 209
Tofu Salad with Nutritional
    Yeast, 203
Tomatillo Guacamole, 207
tomatoes, 7, 9, 84–85, 149, 220
trans fats, 28, 29, 76, 88–89
Truvia, 67
tuna, 40, 41, 42, 43, 205
turbinado sugar, 62
turkey, 33, 38
turkey bacon, 121
turmeric, 70
turnips, 9
24-hour diet makeover
    alcoholic beverages, 174–176
    breakfast, 107–128
    desserts, 176–180
    dinner, 157–173
    lunch, 129–141
    meal plans, 105–106, 223–226
    snacks, 142–156

ultrapasteurization, 17
unfiltered oils, 75
unrefined oils, 75
unrefined salt, 69
unsweetened yogurt, 25
urine tests, 195

vanilla-flavored yogurt, 25
vegetable oil, 71
vegetables
    Asian-style Broccoli Salad, 204

best choices, 7–8
Braised Fennel, 212
breakfast choices, 124–125
canned vegetables, 84–85, 231
cooking tips, 162–165,
    168–169, 233
costs, 6, 8
daily servings, 13, 168–169,
    232
frozen vegetables, 12–13,
    84, 85
Leftover Vegetable Frittata,
    200
lunch recommendations,
    132
nutritional value, 14, 127,
    150, 162–164
organic produce, 9–11
Penne with Sautéed Chard,
    215
Roasted Cauliflower, 211
salad bars, 140–141
seasonality, 8–9
serving quantity, 5–6
shelf-life, 13
shopping tips, 13–14, 227
Silken Asparagus Soup,
    209
snacks, 149–150
Sweet Potato and
    Cauliflower Curry, 210
Tender Kale, 213
Tomatillo Guacamole, 207
washing, 11
vegetarian diets, 159–160
vinaigrette-style dressings, 80
vinegars, 77–80, 230
virgin oils, 75
vitamins
    beef, 33, 34
    cooking method effects,
        162–163
    dairy products, 14, 15, 17
    eggs, 31
    fish, 14
    fruit juice, 32
    health benefits, 181–186
    nondairy milk products, 22
    oatmeal, 57
    pastured meats, 35
    poultry, 33
    produce, 13, 14
    red bell peppers, 6
    timing, 188–189
    vegetables, 150
    vitamin A, 6, 17, 34, 35, 50,
        150, 182
    vitamin B$_{12}$, 33
    vitamin C, 6, 162

vitamin D, 14, 15, 22, 31,
    185–186
vitamin E, 6, 17, 31, 34, 35
vitamin K, 150
vitamin water, 104
wild rice, 50

walnut oil, 71, 76
walnuts, 74, 81
Warm Weather Oats, 199
water
    bottled water, 98–100
    daily servings, 102
    fruit and vitamin waters,
        104
    mineral water, 100
    water filters, 101
water chestnuts, 84
watermelon, 9
weight management
    artificial sweeteners, 65–66
    breakfast, 114–115
    diet trends, 191–196
    late-night snacks, 172–173
    vinegars, 79–80
white beans, 83, 220
whitefish, 40
white meat
    See meat
white mushrooms, 7
white rice, 48
white whole-wheat breads, 56
white whole-wheat flour,
    59
whole food bars, 156
whole-grain foods, 46–47, 51,
    54–56, 59, 127
whole-wheat flour, 59
whole-wheat pastry flour, 59
wild rice, 50
wild salmon, 43
wine, 175, 176
wine vinegar, 78
winter squash, 7, 8, 9, 13
World Health Organization
    (WHO), 177, 178

xylitol, 66

yeast, 203
yellowfin tuna, 40, 42
yogurt, 24–26, 121, 124, 126,
    228

zero-calorie sweeteners
    See artificial
        sweeteners
zinc, 33, 183
zucchini, 9, 149

ABOUT THE AUTHOR

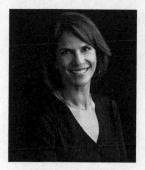 Monica Reinagel, MS, LN, CNS, is the creator of the #1-ranked *Nutrition Diva* podcast and the author of three previous books on health and nutrition. In recent years, she has served as chief nutritionist for NutritionData.com, one of the Internet's leading nutrition information sites, and is a frequent contributor to self.com and Epicurious.com. Monica holds a Master's Degree in Human Nutrition and is a licensed and board-certified nutrition specialist. She received professional culinary training at L'Academie de Cuisine in Washington, D.C. She is a member of the American Dietetic Association, the American College of Nutrition, and the International Association of Culinary Professionals. Monica is also a professional opera singer and has performed with opera companies and orchestras throughout the United States and Germany.

Quick and Dirty Tips™

Helping you do things better.

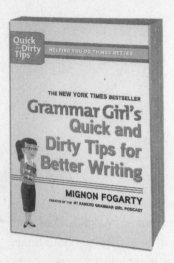

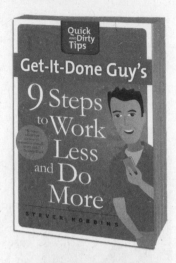

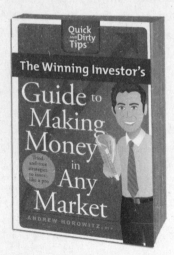

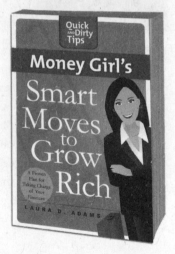